A sensitive, witty, and highly respected psychiatrist, Vicki Berkus, M.D., Ph.D., CEDS, has crafted a pointed ~~ ~ ~ant book about mental fitness—and how to get i+' ~y books on mental health, TEN COMMIT~~ 's addresses the *practical stuff*, the nt need to be mindful of to assure men ~~ alone is simply not enough.

As if she and the reader were havir ~~nversation, Dr. Berkus reminds us to think hard about ~ priorities, our dreams, our feelings, and our relationships. And not to waste a moment in the process! She offers us exercises that are both fun and challenging and fresh questions to ask ourselves and significant others to illuminate a bright path to mental fitness.

With humor, plain talk, practical wisdom, and many examples from her years of practice, Dr. Berkus assures us that we in fact can become mentally fit and add richness and years to our lives.

Roy Erlichman, Ph.D., CEDS
Private Practice
Past President of IAEDP

(International Association of Eating Disorders Professionals) Dr. Erlichman has many years experience as a therapist. He is a dynamic speaker and lectures around the country. His specialty is in eating disorders but his experience is in all areas of psychology.

Dr. Berkus has created a masterpiece for mental fitness. It is a no-nonsense practical approach to becoming and staying mentally healthy and mentally fit.

From the beginning, she challenges you to own your own *stuff* and gives you practical ways to make it happen. This is a must read book for anyone wanting to live fit in a mentally healthy environment.

Mike Kennedy, M.D.
Author of LIVING LEAN
and TEN COMMITMENTS TO BE FOREVER FIT
Chief Medical Officer of Monarch Health Sciences, Inc.
Board certified in Family Practice and Bariatric Medicine

Feeling fit for me has aways started in the home, to help people define their personal space to reflect the brightest aspects of their personalities. TEN COMMITMENTS TO MENTAL FITNESS teaches the most important lesson of all—how to be mentally fit, allowing the true beauty of their personalities shine brighter then ever.

—Nate Berkus, author of HOME RULES

Dr. Berkus proves that if we really want to live a life that honors our deepest desires, we CAN make it happen—it all starts in the mind. Yes, it takes deep commitment, but we are worth it; and her book makes the work easier and the journey more enjoyable!

—Andrea Pennington, M.D., C.Ac.
President, Pennington Institute for Health & Wellness
Author of THE PENNINGTON PLAN, 5 SIMPLE STEPS FOR ACHIEVING VIBRANT HEALTH, SPIRITUAL GROWTH AND EMOTIONAL WELLBEING

TEN COMMITMENTS TO MENTAL FITNESS

by
Vicki Berkus, M.D., Ph.D., CEDS

Robert D. Reed Publishers • Bandon, OR

Robert D. Reed Publishers
P.O. Box 1992
Bandon, OR 97411
Phone: 541-347-9882 • Fax: -9883
E-mail: 4bobreed@msn.com
web site: www.rdrpublishers.com

Typesetter: **Barbara Kruger**
Cover Designer: **Grant Prescott**
Editor: **Cleone Lyvonne**

ISBN 1-931741-61-1

Library of Congress Control Number 2005902921

Manufactured, typeset and printed in the United States of America

This book is dedicated to
my parents,
Bea and Carl Berkus,
who taught me
the meaning of unconditional love.

Contents

Preface

Accept the Challenge to Change,
and Become Mentally Fit

TEN COMMITMENTS TO MENTAL FITNESS will improve your mental fitness by helping you understand some of the same principles that can be learned in psychotherapy. Experts have provided an abundance of information about how to attain physical fitness, and most of us already know how to eat healthy foods, exercise, and stop smoking and drinking. However, many people do not know how to improve their mental fitness. TEN COMMITMENTS TO MENTAL FITNESS provides answers; and it will empower readers to have the courage to examine their mental fitness, learn how to identify and keep behaviors that makes sense, and let go of behaviors that do not.

The Ten Commitments outlined by Dr. Berkus are about learning to put yourself first, taking responsibility for your feelings, setting priorities, and being honest with yourself. She challenges you to ask some very direct questions that can only be answered by looking inward. After assessing where you are in the present, you can move forward with changes that will improve your life. The Commitments also ask you to examine your relationships, because good mental fitness includes cultivating relationships with people who honor each other's boundaries.

Many people struggle because they have lost their connection to spirituality, relationships, and the things in nature or the arts that they value. Reconnection can be realized by the examination of *self-talk*, which fills our minds and seems to come automatically.

Negative self-talk can result in destructive behaviors and cause us to criticize those who are trying to help. These feelings can affect our bodies, resulting in headaches, digestive upset, pain, weakness, insomnia, or fatigue. The commitment to understanding the mind-body connection can free you to take action and overcome physical symptoms.

The challenge presented in TEN COMMITMENTS TO MENTAL FITNESS is realizing that your present way of life may not be working, and that you can take a different, more positive course of action. Put yourself first and become mentally fit.

Vicki Berkus, M.D., Ph.D., CEDS, is a member of the the Monarch Health Sciences Medical Board. She consults with coaches in addressing various psychological aspects of healthy eating. Dr. Berkus has written several articles on obesity, and writes and speaks for Monarch on mental health issues. She is the immediate past president of the International Association of Eating Disorders Professionals and speaks to physicians, therapists, and nutritionists in order to increase their awareness of the severity of eating disorders

Dr. Berkus is a regular contributor to *Connections*, the publication for the organization IAEDP. She received a Master's degree from the University of Nevada–Reno, a Ph.D. in biochemistry from Oklahoma State University, and an M.D. from the University of Oklahoma, School of Medicine.

Dr. Berkus completed a psychiatry residency at the University of Arizona, College of Medicine. She is board-certified in Psychiatry and Neurology. Her advanced certification (CEDS) is from the IAEDP program. She has headed an in-patient eating disorders program for eight years and is currently in private practice in Tucson, Arizona.

Introduction

Most people are tuned into the concept of physical fitness and could describe several plans to help them *get fit*. I wondered if it would be as easy to come up with a plan for mental fitness. I decided to write the book to help people who have never really made the commitment to improve their mental health. I see a lot of morbidity (consequences associated with poor decisions whether it is involving social, financial, spiritual, interpersonal, or family of origin issues.)

The idea of committing yourself to anything usually involves a payoff. What's in it for me? Well, I will ask you one question: "Is your way working?" If it is, you should feel *good enough* about yourself at the end of the day—about your thoughts, your decisions, your health, and your relationships.

People come to see me because their way isn't working and they don't know what to do. This can result in depression, anxiety, sleeplessness, weight gain or loss, and a lot of pain, both mentally and physically.

After working with patients in an in-patient setting, I would frequently hear: "Dr. Berkus, being here for 30 days is like being in weekly therapy for three years!" The message was that if they took time out of their lives for 30 days and really made a commitment to mental fitness, it paid off.

Most people can't afford the luxury of a 30-day in-patient program, but being human, we all have interpersonal relationship issues, grief and loss issues, spiritual issues, self-esteem issues, and family of origin issues. We tend to stuff them, avoid them, ruminate, intellectualize, rationalize and a number of other behaviors to keep functioning. It's not that most of us wouldn't like to put some sort of resolution to these problems, but we don't have the tools to do so.

How many of you have started a diet on a Monday, full of commitment, resolve, and determination, only to decide by Wednesday that it isn't that crucial; and you will just *watch* it and start again when you aren't dealing with _____ _____ (fill in the blank)? Did any of us have classes in making commitments and keeping them? I doubt it.

This book deals with increasing your awareness of everyday behaviors and the consequences they bring. It offers options to try and challenges you to keep what works and let go of what doesn't. If you start to have feelings about something in the book, then chances are that it fits, and you may want to commit to new behaviors.

My favorite mantra to my patients is: "You don't have to like it, you don't even have to want it, but you're going to do it because deep down inside, you know it's the right thing to do."

You made the first commitment: you picked up this book and are thinking about how it might apply or help you. Good job! Now the work begins.

Be not afraid of growing slowly;
be afraid only of standing still.
—Chinese Proverb

Chapter 1

Commitment to Know I Count

**You must be the change
you wish to see in the world.**
—Mahatma Gandhi

Mary sat down and started to cry. Going for the affect, I asked her what the tears were about, and she started to complain that her boyfriend chose to go to a sporting event with his pals instead of spending her birthday with her. She was hurt and angry. She did admit that she had told him to go, it was no big deal, and they would celebrate at another time. So the next question was, "Why did you tell him it was OK?"

She responded that he had done this in the past and didn't expect it to be a problem. She was sending mixed signals so I asked her, "What do you really need from him in this relationship?"

She looked at me with a puzzled expression on her face and asked, "What do you mean?"

I again repeated, "What do you need in this relationship?"

The answer I received from her (and numerous patients before her) was, "I don't know."

My typical response is: "If you don't know what you need, then how do you expect him to know? Is he a mind reader?"

She smiled and said "no" and we started to work on helping her define her needs.

Whether it is with a spouse, parent, boss, friend, pet, etc., how often do you sit down and think about what you need in a relationship? We rarely take the time to evaluate ourselves on a daily basis. The norm is to hurry through the morning and start the tasks for the day.

It is interesting to me that if I ask people who are in their second or third marriages how they define their needs, it seems that they have learned when to make something an issue or a need and when to keep quiet. We laugh together that if their spouse only knew some of their unsaid thoughts, things would heat up quickly.

The idea is that we can identify our feelings or responses to others and yet not react to them in a way that may perpetrate our loved ones. One way to do this is to understand how you are doing on a given day and take that into consideration before you interact with others. This next exercise will help you get to that point.

Daily Psychological Inventory

I had a mentor in medical school that challenged us as medical students to do a **Daily Psychological Inventory**. We looked at him with our typical "yah, right—in our spare time" expressions. Not until after my residency in psychiatry did I realize how important this exercise could be, especially if you are the type of person who puts the needs of others first. The Inventory consists of asking yourself four questions and writing the answers down for the first week. They are as follows:

1. **How do I feel about me today? (Remember to use only feelings.)**

   _____

2. **How do I feel about the significant others in my life?**

   _____

3. How do I feel about today's tasks?

_____

4. How do I feel about yesterday's events?

_____

Question 1: How do I feel about me today? (Remember to use only feelings.) How many times do you look at yourself in the mirror and are aware of your feelings? I work with patients struggling with eating disorders—anorexia, bulimia and compulsive overeating. "I feel fat" is a common statement. I'll respond with: "*Fat* isn't a feeling, so if you substitute a feeling for the word *fat*, what would it be?" The most common answers are disgust, fear, hate, loathing, and anger. Now I know that there is work to be done.

If your answer is close to one of the above answers (disgust, hate, etc.), then it is your job to deal with your feelings **before** you start your day.

Do you ever stop to consider why some mornings are *good* and others are *bad*? Why is it you can just hop out of bed some days, and others, you first run through a list of possible excuses of why you may just stay in bed? If these examples have hit home, you may decide to journal, check in with a therapist, or ask yourself what just happened. Did you have a particular memory or feeling? Is that your usual way to start your day?

Yes, I know mornings can be hectic, and you may get some strange looks if you begin talking to yourself in the mirror. Yet, taking a few moments for you can resolve some anger or sadness. Can you see how much energy it can take to hold onto those feelings? This *holding on may cause you to miss other options for your day.*

Question 2: How do I feel about the significant others in my life? When you ask yourself about significant others in your life, you may be surprised who pops into your head. Is it a friend, relative, boss, or coworker? What do you need to do about those feelings? Is just being aware of them enough?

If you decide that you feel hatred for your boss and this happens on most mornings, you can ignore it and continue to be angry. (Is that how you want to be remembered—as an angry person?) Or you may decide to act on your feelings. Is it time to change jobs, have a talk with your boss, or get help to deal with the anger?

If the same person keeps coming into your thoughts, is that person contributing to your life or do you need to end the relationship? "Darn so-and-so said he would call last night and let me know if I had to pick up something for the morning. He never does what he says he will do!" Well, if you knew that, why are you still expecting him to follow through on what he says? Could you have called him or set it up that if you didn't hear from him by 10:00 p.m., you would pick up the items and see him at the meeting? This way, you are not waiting for someone else to behave in a certain manner.

If a workman, barber, or manicurist is always late, or is doing poor work or gets too needy; do you need to end the relationship? When you take the time to look at how you feel about the people in your life, you may make some changes that can really make life simpler. If everyone is getting to you, then it may be *your stuff*, not everyone around you. Read on.

Question 3: How do I feel about today's tasks? If I look at my schedule and my response is "Oh, crap!"—it isn't about the schedule. That's *my stuff*. I know what my days are usually like, and if that is my reaction on a particular day, I need to figure out what is going on *with me* before I start my day. I know that I will see patients, maybe give a talk, and make some calls. What is going on today that makes those things seem overwhelming? It may take a few minutes to figure it out on any given day. Was I irritated when I woke up? Did I put off something that was going to make my schedule more hectic? Am I overtired? Am I catching something? I may need a way to measure my irritability such as the following example.

Did you ever notice your own behavior around hitting red lights? Some days it doesn't seem to matter, and you are OK with listening to your favorite radio station. Then there are those days when you are convinced that if you *just killed* the driver in front of you, you wouldn't miss another red light. It isn't about the driver or the red light: it's about what is going on with you. It helps to pick your *barometer* to help you check in with yourself. Is it red lights or how you respond to being put *on hold* when you are making calls? Pick something.

One factor to look at is the importance of anniversary reactions. This particular mentor who challenged us to do this **Daily Psychological Inventory** was aware of feeling extremely sad while doing his inventory one day and couldn't put his finger on the cause. After thinking about it, he realized it was the anniversary of the death of a good friend and mentor. He decided to cancel his appointments and go pay his respects at the gravesite. He honored his feelings and knew his limitations.

If I feel that my reaction to my schedule ("Oh, crap!") really needs an intervention, I may decide to cancel some of my appointments and go see my therapist, or add some down time for a quick walk—whatever works.

Question 4: How do I feel about yesterday's events? Use this question to check in with yourself and see what emotional baggage you are still carrying around with you. Are you still angry with someone, disappointed, or sad? What do you need to do about it? How are you going to put some sort of resolution to those feelings? Would you want your surgeon or your psychiatrist to be hanging onto anger that they experienced the day before? (*I don't think so.*)

Are you the type of person who has to run the previous day through your head and decide if you did the right thing, or said the right thing? What would you need to do to *quiet the judge* and let yesterday be *good enough*? Just the exercise of checking in with yourself lets your subconscious know that *you count, your feelings count, and your thoughts count.*

I challenge you to try out the **Daily Psychological Inventory** and write down your answers for the first week. After that, you can make it a habit by running through the questions in your mind while you're doing your morning routine. The purpose of this exercise is to help you get in touch with your feelings and to help your sub-conscious learn: *"You count, your feelings count, and your thoughts count!"*

I have had patients tell me what they are *thinking* when I ask the proverbial psychiatrist's question: "How did that *feel?*" I will let them finish their thought and ask again: "How did that *feel?*" Sometimes this will go on four or five times before they realize how difficult it was for them to get in touch with the feelings—not the thoughts. I even give some patients a *cheat sheet* of little faces portraying different feelings. They can scan the sheet and pick which feelings are the ones they are experiencing.

A patient told me, "I never get angry."

I said, "Really! How does that happen? What do you do with your anger?"

"I don't know," she said. "My friends say that I am the most even-tempered person they know, and they have never seen me angry."

Meanwhile, I'm thinking that showing anger and feeling anger are two different things. Many of my patients will tell me they will do just about anything to avoid conflict. Usually I will do my best over the next few sessions to allow the person to get angry. The anger is there, usually masked as another feeling.

Did you ever notice that when some women get angry, they cry? It's not unusual for women to confuse the two feelings. They may have learned that tears are allowed but not a show of anger. Disagreeing or correcting someone resulted in being hit or banished from the room. Kids who had parents who were alcoholics or prone to rage learn to hide their anger very well, sometimes even from themselves.

I grew up in a time when the *"kids should be seen and not heard"* saying was in vogue. There were times when the kids were always excluded from the adults, and it was not OK to interrupt because you were having certain feelings. I remember having friends and never being with their parents or getting to know their parents. The idea was that parents put food on the table and a roof over their heads: that is what parents do. Rarely did both parents come to school carnivals or programs. Letting others know your feelings was not something that was taught. Therapy or visits to a psychiatrist were only for those who were having *a nervous breakdown.* Many of my patients never knew what a school counselor was or had access to one. This was not a time that was conducive to discussing feelings. So how do you teach the concept of discussing your feelings if it is a foreign behavior to you? You don't. You focus instead on the external things in life.

Too often we get caught up in the external things in our life, and it becomes the "grocery-shopping counts" or "balancing-the-budget counts" or "what-I'm-wearing counts" or "how-my-body-looks counts." Get the picture? The concept of *"I count"* only hits home when we feel in danger or have to come to the aid of someone.

Any mother (or father) who has dealt with a sick child who depends on her to survive has realized her decisions or feelings *count.* She may demand to see a doctor immediately or insist on staying in the hospital with her child. It is almost automatic how clear her needs become apparent. It only takes one near-death experience, and suddenly you realize that *small things don't seem to* **count** *as much anymore.*

Why wait until a crisis forces you to become aware that *you count, your needs count, and your feelings count*?

Picture the person you want to be with because you respect, trust and value his/her opinion or feedback. You will drop most things to be with that person—right? You've decided that his/her presence is a priority in your life.

Why shouldn't that person be you???? I don't mean it in a narcissistic selfish way, but it is OK to demonstrate a *healthy selfishness* and be in touch with your feelings at any given time. I'm asking you to go inward to find a sense of well-being instead of looking externally (to a friend, spouse, situation, or drug). It's a hard way to go through life if you feel that your needs aren't being met.

Couples come in for therapy; and nine times out of ten, the major complaint is that one partner feels s/he are carrying the load and his/her needs aren't being met in the relationship. This is usually the case when one partner is in a professional school where s/he has to be on call or study for boards. The *other partner* becomes *infantilized.* This means s/he is expected to follow orders such as: "I have to work so you need to pick up the cleaning" or "Take Mom to the doctor" or "Plan the party." It's not that one partner is more child-like (infant), but s/he is the one with the time and ability to carry out the household tasks. This is OK until the professional finishes and the spouse now demands: "Now it's my turn." More divorces happen because one person's needs aren't met in the relationship. It has been a parent/child relationship. Then when one partner insists the relationship become adult-to-adult, the other person, in their anger, gets global and accuses: "You always, never…, etc." This escalates because one person hasn't had his/her needs met for a long time.

News Flash

IT'S NO ONE ELSE'S JOB
TO TAKE CARE OF YOUR FEELINGS!

When a patient describes a situation and out come the words, "She made me so angry!" I want to ask, "How did she do that? Did she hold a gun to your head and demand that you get angry or kiss your life goodbye?"

We all have choices on how to react to what others are doing, thinking, saying or feeling. If a patient walks into my office and is late, do I have a choice of how to react?

• Sure! I can get into my *angry kid* and yell: "How do you expect me to see my other patients on time if you are late?"

• OR I could choose to act like a *punitive parent* and say: "You knew what time your appointment was! You'll have to reschedule. I can't see you now."

• OR I could choose to be a *nurturing parent* and say, "Please have a seat and take a deep breath. We can deal with this. No one died so let's put this in perspective."

The problem starts when we *react* instead of *taking action*. If we stopped and considered our choices, chances are we would make better decisions.

You ask, "What decisions?"

Did you ever have a relationship in which the other person had NO OPINIONS! "Where do you want to eat?" Answer: "I don't care." "What movie do you want to see?" Answer: "I don't care." The message they are sending is YOU **COUNT**, I DON'T. After awhile, you just want to shake or strangle them, yelling, "MAKE A DECISION!!!"

How about the person who calls you and comes from I **COUNT**, YOU DON'T? A conversation may start: "I'm busy so I can only talk for a minute. Will you pick up my favorite Chinese food on your way home, and I'll pay you back next week? By the way, I invited a friend to eat with us; and I know you hate him, but be nice—OK? I may be late, but I'll be too busy to call so just expect me when you see me. Bye!"

How were you feeling while you were reading this? Angry? Does this scenario remind you of anyone in your life? Do you put up with this kind of behavior?

Let's look at this scenario from an *I COUNT, YOU COUNT* position. Your friend calls and asks what you want to do about dinner. You respond, "I would like either Chinese or Italian." You both decide that it is your turn to pick it up, and you'll collect her share of the cost when you meet. She lets you know that her friend (who she knows you don't like) may show up; and that if it happens, she will go out with that person for dessert and give you an *easy out*. It feels better, doesn't it?

So, how do you listen to your feelings and decide what behaviors trigger reactions in you and which are OK? We're back to the needs list, and if you don't know what your needs are, no one else will! The second important part of getting your needs met by others is to choose those people who can meet those needs.

Frequently I will hear from a patient that one of her parents was never emotionally available to her. She was never hugged or told: "I love you." So here she is as an adult, and whom do you think she is complaining about in terms of not getting her emotional needs met? You got it—the parent!

Looking at the patient, who may be in her 20s or 30s, I will ask her if she expects her parent to suddenly change, and she always tells me "no." She doesn't *get it* that it's *her stuff* and not the parent who has been sending the same signals throughout the patient's life. She keeps going back to the same person to try to get her needs met, and it just won't happen. We will then work together to help that patient understand that she needs to look elsewhere, preferably inward, but maybe to a group or a therapist. The patient may need to do some grief work around not having two nurturing parents to help her feel that *she counted*.

This may be one reason it is so hard to lose a parent—no one has ever had that kind of ability to help you feel that **YOU COUNT**. When you create the belief that **YOU COUNT**, then good feelings will naturally follow your positive thought patterns. Then when you learn to speak clearly to others about your needs and boundaries, your new **I-COUNT** actions will pay off in all of your relationships.

Since I work with many patients who "hate their bodies" and struggle with food, I try to help them understand why they are behaving from the premise that FOOD COUNTS and not them. We try to understand the power that they give to food: how they perceive it one minute as a best friend, and the next, as an enemy that has more control than they do.

It is easy to understand why they are exhausted, depressed, frustrated and hopeless when you consider the amount of energy that goes into thinking about food: verbally punishing themselves after eating, shopping, eating in secret, focusing on the parts of their bodies that they hate, etc. Their WEIGHT COUNTS and becomes their priority over their life. I have patients who are absolutely sure that if the number on the scale is not what they expect, it will be a *bad day*. They may then choose to binge or restrict their food. They have given the number on the scale their power, and the consequences will usually include negative self-talk.

Since Jane was a little girl, the message she received was "Be a good girl and _____." The blank might be filled in with "Get daddy his paper" or "Help mommy set the table" or "Take care of your little brother." She started in her role of caretaker very early.

She came in for treatment of her eating disorder. She was also involved with food from an early age (shopping with mom, pushing the miniature shopping cart, cooking, etc.) and also learned to use food to self-soothe. She didn't understand that her anxiety was based on not getting her needs met. She was so used to stuffing her feelings and being watchful of others that she had no idea how to do the same thing for herself. She married someone who had a lot of needs and looked to her to fill most of them. Her children were also demanding and had learned that mom would handle things.

We had to go back to square one and help her identify her feelings and give her tools to realize that she couldn't be everything to everyone.

She eventually learned to give herself permission to put herself first and decide that *she counted* just as much as the ones she loved. Once she started to *value herself,* she was able to take charge of her life and her feelings. She started to lose weight, feel in control and enjoy her life!

When teens are angry about being grounded or want more privileges, their assignment is to write down a list of things that are good in their lives. Many cannot make the leap from focusing on want they can't do as opposed to all the things they can do that bring pleasure to their lives. The external things begin to COUNT such as a later curfew, more allowance, hanging out with the friends they want to, using drugs, and being cool. The task of helping them look inward can be tedious, but it can lead to more positive attitudes and behaviors. Remember, teens seem to be in the moment, and they need to learn how to stop and consider the *big picture.*

Whether you are a teen, a young adult, middle aged, or a senior, there is no time like the present moment to **commit to put yourself first, identify your needs, and know that you count**. On-going self-awareness to this first commitment is part of a life-long process *to be mentally fit*. It does take time to work on these new behaviors, but you will get out of the work what you put into it.

Remember, *you count, your thoughts count, and your feelings count.*

Chapter 2

Commitment to
Take Responsibility for My Feelings

**Of all knowledge
the wise and good seek most
to know themselves.**
—William Shakespeare, British playwright (1564-1616)

Now that you are starting to get in touch with your feelings (by doing the **Daily Psychological Inventory**), it is now time to learn to take responsibility for those feelings. There are three basic steps to doing this, as follows:

Step 1: Identify the intensity of your feelings.

Step 2. Own your feelings.

Step 3. Take action: deal with your feelings and provide a healthy resolution to those feelings.

Let's look at these steps in more detail.

Step 1: Identify the intensity of your feelings.

\ Picture a ski slope with the top of the slope,
\ the plateau representing *rage*.
\ As you start down the ski slope, you get a third of
\ the way down and hit *anger*.
\ At the halfway point is *frustration*.
\ At the bottom of the hill is *annoyance*.

Are you the type of person who starts up the slope (forget the skiing) and goes from annoyance to rage in a flash? Do you manage to keep most things at the annoyance level?

EXERCISE: Draw your own ski slope and figure out where you hang most of the time.

If your biggest problem is to go from the annoyance level to the frustrated level pretty quickly, then put some stairs between the two and decide what interventions or actions you need to take to keep things at the annoyance level.

Do you need to journal, take a time out, break whatever is getting you upset into parts, or get help (novel idea for a lot of *"I can do it myself"* people)? Let's look at an example: you come home, open the fridge, and reach for something when an open can of flat soda tips over and spills its contents all over the fridge and the floor. Where would you be?

- Is this an annoyance that you can smile at and know that you DID IT AGAIN?

- Or do the next words out of your mouth need to be censored?

Are you going to hold on to the anger until they (husband, wife, son, daughter, etc.) get home, or can you let it go? If you can't, then start writing down the alternatives to holding the anger.

1. Do you stop buying cans and go to bottles?

2. Do you put a sticky note on the fridge? Maybe it says, "If the can is open, finish it! Do not put it back in the fridge."

3. Do you put a sign in the fridge: "All cans go in the door only?"

What do these three actions have in common? You are changing your behavior and not expecting others to change theirs at that minute. Sure, you could argue that you now expect other people in your home to honor the signs. The point is that you took your anger and put some sort of resolution to it. If the signs don't work, you may decide to throw out open cans the minute you get home. It is YOUR ACTION and YOUR BEHAVIOR. Depending on others to change their behavior is a set up. You learn to pick your battles and let go of a lot of them.

My personal favorite scenario is to walk into the kitchen and see dirty items or wrappers on the counter when the dishwasher and the trash can are only two feet from the area. My choice: do I decide to keep it to the annoyance level and put them where they belong or do I rush up to rage so fast that I want to throw the dishes or take the wrappers and the garbage and toss them in the offender's room? (In some homes, this is the first step to a domestic violence charge.) Feelings can escalate quickly in some environments. Pick an example you frequently encounter, and check out where you are on your scale. Do you need to do some work?

NOTE: You can apply this same system of identifying the intensity of your feelings with any feelings: guilt, shame, sadness/depression, remorse, hate, etc.

Step 2. Own your feelings.

The hardest feelings to deal with are shame and guilt. If you have a dog, watch his expression if he has piddled in the house and you exclaim: "What did you do?" Most dogs will cower. Right? Or look away.

Try to remember an incident in which you felt shamed. Did you wet the bed or get caught in a lie? As an adult, did you eat something you *shouldn't* have or have an affair?

The feelings just happen. We all use certain defenses, whether it is to blame someone else or joke about the incident. It takes courage to own your feelings and learn to resolve them in a healthy way. It's much easier to resort to a defense than to sit in the feelings (IT DOESN'T FEEL GOOD) and own them.

Many compulsive overeaters will tell me that they eat to *numb* their feelings; and if they focus on the food, they can decrease the intensity of their feelings. They are the first to admit that they are not hungry when they eat, but that they are angry, scared, or ashamed of their size. Then the vicious circle of behavior gets started: eat, feel guilty, and eat more to numb the feelings rather than owning them.

The same things apply to people who gamble, drink, use relationships, or any of the other numerous addictive behaviors. They can't tolerate the feelings that occur. The idea then is to deal with feelings as they come up—not stuff them until they are addressed at another time, or come out sideways or unintentionally in a dramatic way.

Do you ever get angry at work, but instead of addressing your anger, come home and yell at the kids or the dog? Welcome to the human race. Displaced anger is another defense mechanism against the anger felt initially. How many times do you try to make amends to someone by saying, "I'm not angry with you; it's just that so and so happened, and I can't help my anger?" Yes, you can. You can own it, go back to your chart, and look at your interventions.

If you are in a situation and are aware that you are annoyed, can you address the situation at that level? For example, what if you are standing in line at the grocery store and are in a hurry when the lady in front of you pulls out 50 coupons? Do you have a choice of how to respond? Of course! Here are just a few of the many options you could do, each one demonstrating a different level of intensity in your feelings:

- Say something really brash like: "Hey, lady, what the hell are you doing?"

- Say something snippy out loud to the woman with the coupons like: "Couldn't you get organized before you got to the cashier? People are held up because of you!"

- Roll your eyes and mutter, thereby letting people around you know that you are not happy.

Or, you can own your feelings (anger, frustration, impatience) and...

- Either change lanes or read a few more headlines of the magazines at the checkout counter.

- *Breathe* or calm yourself down by describing your environment to yourself as if you were describing it to an individual who was blind.

- Look at the lady with compassion and say to yourself, "Just like me, this lady is trying to do things in a hurry and didn't take time to get organized. Just like me, this lady…"

- Silently in your head, repeat to yourself the lyrics to a favorite song.

The brain has a difficult time hanging on to two thoughts at a time. To take responsibility for your feelings (and consequently your behaviors), you would have to let go of all the negative thoughts you were having about this woman and her coupons.

A great place to look at people and their behaviors is at a crowded airport. What a great place to practice keeping things at the annoyance level and not letting them get to a frustration level. Your plane is delayed or the security line gets held up. Do you let yourself get frustrated, jump in the global arena and say: "This *always* happens" or "I *never* get a break!"

The jump into a victim role can be all too familiar. "Why me?" Many times, it's easier to jump into the victim role and blame others for your feelings ("THE SECURITY PEOPLE MADE ME MAD!") rather than own your feelings and ask yourself, "Why am I taking this personally and getting so angry?"

It may take therapy to learn the ability to take responsibility for your feelings and be able to tell yourself: "OK. This is life. Why am I acting this way?"

Is this the behavior that was modeled for you as a kid? The continued crescendo up to the anger level can happen so fast for some people that they are acting on their anger before they know it—slamming a door, demanding to see *someone in charge* or feeling an increased heart rate or blood pressure. Do they stop and look around and ask themselves, "Why isn't everyone around me just as angry?" No. They are on the way up to rage as if on automatic pilot.

This is really about a real or perceived loss of control. Most people—who have problems with anger, whether it is road rage, judgmental thinking, or verbal abuse—may have to learn the tools to control their anger. I often tell parents to keep a lot of phone books around and give them to their kids to rip up when they are angry. Wouldn't it be great if there were punching bags located in airports? Sadly, some people would just escalate more.

It isn't wrong or bad to have feelings. Welcome again to the human race. It's what you do with the feelings that can cause consequences.

Jack was the CEO of a company and was used to having his needs met when requested. His father had been in the military and was an alcoholic who was verbally and physically abusive to his family. Jack had reported feeling helpless around protecting his mother from his father. He mainly tried to anticipate his father's moods and would be as inconspicuous as possible. The message he perceived was "You don't count."

He came in for help because his wife had threatened to leave him unless he "got help with his anger." They had been at their favorite restaurant, and Jack's dinner was cold when it arrived. He became angry and verbally abusive towards the waiter. He was unable to calm down even when the owner offered to intervene and take the charge off for his dinner. He stormed out of the restaurant and told his wife to follow him. He then proceeded to back into a parked car in his rush to get out of the parking lot. She did not speak to him for the next two days and finally told him to get help or she would ask him to move out.

Jack sat with his arms and legs crossed (closed position) and informed me that he thought shrinks were just into a lot of psychobabble, and he was only here to keep his wife quiet. He thought that she overreacted and was making a mountain out of a molehill. He assured me that he wanted to stay in the marriage.

We started to talk about his anger and he was able to see that it also spilled over into the workplace. He perceived that people avoided him and just kept their interactions at a minimum. He was able to identify with how they might be feeling.

He agreed to keep another appointment and to think about how he might have handled the episode at the restaurant differently.

His process had started.

When patients come in and I ask them what were the rules around having feelings when they were young, I frequently hear that showing their feelings wasn't allowed. Phrases like "don't be a baby," "don't be a bother," or "don't be angry" were common. Unfortunately, kids hear "don't be" which is pretty hard to hear at any age. The other classic phrase was: "You want something to cry about, then I'll give you something to cry about!"

I'm not blaming parents; it is more about how society treats people who express their feelings. "Real men don't cry." "Real ladies don't get angry."

I once watched the interchange between a little seven-year-old girl as she forgave her daddy for yelling at her when he had been drinking. He was in a recovery program, and part of their family process was to really listen to each other's confrontations and to make amends. He was in tears, and the connection between the two after he owned his feelings (shame, sadness, guilt) was touching and inspiring. He made his commitment to her to stop his anger before the yelling stage.

Three of the most powerful words in our language are "I am sorry." Most people will respond to you owning your feelings. Maybe this commitment should be standard for all people who pass from their teens to adulthood.

We all have these feelings, and learning to deal with them as they come up instead of stuffing them is important. So here are a few tips.

1. **Recognize that your thoughts create your feelings, and you can change your thoughts.**

2. **Based on your thoughts, you can decide to choose a behavior conducive to feeling good after you have taken action.** *(Read on.)*

Step 3. Take action: deal with your feeling and provide a healthy resolution to those feelings.

How often do you confront someone on his or her behavior? If a friend tells a racist joke, the usual response is to hold your feelings in instead of letting the person know that when they told the joke, you felt angry or fearful. Those feeling don't just go away. When you confront someone, the goal is to own and take care of your feelings—not to expect the other person to change. You can't control someone else's thoughts, feelings, actions—only your own. It takes courage to look at the offender and say: "When you told the joke, I felt angry or embarrassed" (or whatever the feeling was). You are not judging—just expressing your feelings. Chances are high that you will feel better when you speak up for yourself respectfully. If the other person then chooses to apologize, and/or stop before they open their mouth next time, that's a bonus.

It is hard to own your behavior and to make amends if that behavior has affected someone else. We are human and will say or do things that affect others. If we do this out of anger, fear, boredom, or loneliness, we are the only ones who can take responsibility and model a new behavior for others by apologizing, learning from our mistakes, and not doing *whatever* again.

"I'm not angry; I'm disappointed." Was that a parent comment or what? Wouldn't you have rather have heard the anger? This is one of the hardest commitments for most people. "*They made me* so angry, *it made me* so angry, *the dumb machine made me* so angry, *the song made me* sad." The *made me's* are rampant in our vocabulary. The ability to change it to "I felt angry when the machine didn't respond" takes you out of the victim role.

My patients who are trying to control their weight frequently tell me that they were doing well until someone *made them mad*. They were hurt by what someone said, or they didn't get the job they were hoping for, and they said, "Screw it!" Then they binged. The ability to pause and do a reality-check with themselves or others takes practice. It is much easier to *react* than to take *action*.

An exercise that I suggest is that they sit down and list 10 things they can do when they get angry instead of eat. Remember, I'm not saying, "DON'T GET ANGRY!" It's human to get angry; it's what you do with the anger that's the focus of this chapter. In order to *take responsibility for your feelings*, the commitment in this chapter, you need to transform out of your negative feelings so that your behaviors make you feel better, not compound your negative feelings.

I'm back to the stance: "There is no gun at your head *making you stay in your anger*. You choose to because it is comfortable." I'm not saying it feels good, but it is a familiar behavior. We all know the consequences when we lose control—shame, guilt, weight gain, feeling out of control—but these are predictable, and in that sense there is comfort.

It is the unknown that brings the uncomfortable feeling and the *dis-ease*. I tell my patients that if they change their behaviors, it *should* feel uncomfortable—it's new, it's different—but it can become a good habit.

Remember the first time you got behind the wheel of a car, and it felt overwhelming? How hard do you hit the gas? How far do you turn the wheel? When do you start the turn and when do you check the mirrors? "DON'T TALK TO ME—I'M DRIVING!" It is almost hard to believe that something that is so natural now was so overwhelming at the beginning. The same thing applies to owning our feelings and taking action around them instead of reacting.

EXERCISE: List 10 things you can do with your anger.

1. _____

2. _____

3. _____

4. _____

5. _____

6. _____

7. _____

8. _____

9. _____

10. _____

NOTE: You can make lists to deal with any feelings that cause you distress: guilt, shame, sadness/depression, remorse, hate, etc.

Taking responsibility for your feelings may mean apologizing to someone, writing a letter, or doing something to address your feelings, such as therapy, joining a support group, talking with clergy, or seeing your physician. The nice thing about being an adult is that we can re-decide things. We don't have to listen to *old tapes* that go on in our heads, whether they were messages from parents, significant others, or people who pretended to be friends. We can re-decide to change how we respond to certain situations and take charge of our feelings.

You may get to the point where you can do some healthy bragging about the good feelings you are having! It's OK.

Commit yourself to take responsibility for your feelings to be mentally fit by following these steps:

1. Be aware of the intensity of your feelings.

2. Own your feelings.

3. Take action to resolve them.

Chapter 3

Commitment to Set Priorities in My Life

People with goals succeed
Because they know where they're going.
—Earl Nightingale, American businessman (1921-1989)

A patient of mine had been late for his last three appointments, and I asked him, "If I told you that I would give you a million dollars to be on time for your next appointment, would you find a way to do it?"

He grinned and said, "Probably."

I challenged him: "PROBABLY????"

He was able to laugh and assured me he would find a way.

It's all about priorities. If you stop and look at your accomplishments in your life, then ask yourself, "How did I make that happen?" Whether it was your education, your selection of a spouse, a career, or an original piece of work—what was it that allowed you to make it a priority? If that concept is too overwhelming, ask yourself how you passed a test or paid a bill on time. Some reasoning allowed you to complete a task. Is it a pattern for you? Do you tend to procrastinate until you are down to the wire and then rise to the occasion, or do you prioritize the things you want to get done in life and systematically address them?

Priorities are met, to name a few reasons, out of obligation, fear, desire to obtain financial success or personal recognition. Some people will tell you it was sheer determination, but something deeper was behind the determination. Was it a need to finish what was started? Finishing my doctorate was pure endurance: it was a decision to finish what was started.

Some of my patients wish they could experience OCD (obsessive-compulsive disorder) for a month. Those of you that have it are probably angry or confused right now, but it isn't that they are demeaning the seriousness of the disease. It means that they are clueless about how to set their priorities and make them happen. Face it. Sticking with something usually means keeping your focus. This is especially hard for adults who have ADD (Attention Deficit Disorder). They start several projects but just can't seem to complete them.

Think about what gets in your way when you decide to complete a goal. List the three biggest stumbling blocks.

1. _____

2. _____

3. _____

Did you put *time, money, support from family* or *significant other*? Do these tend to change, or do they stay pretty consistent? How could you try to change your behavior to sidestep one of these blocks?

I have had overweight patients wish for a short bout of anorexia. It is out of desperation that these ideas even come up. How many times have you started a diet on a Monday with the best of intentions and by Wednesday, you have decided that you don't look that bad and you will start another time? Do you talk yourself out of your goals over and over?

Start making short-term goals that are easily obtainable. When you feel confident that you can start fulfilling these, then move to intermediate goals and then onto long-term goals.

List two short-term goals that are manageable.

1. _____

2. _____

The idea is to meet these and start to build your confidence so you can continue to do this with little effort. For example, finish reading this chapter today, complete the fill-ins, and give yourself a compliment and/or pat on the back. Now you have reached your short-term goal. Next, for your intermediate goal, commit to reading the whole book by a certain date. For your long-term goal, focus on becoming mentally fit and commit to changing your behaviors.

There may be many goals we have for ourselves, but how we prioritize those goals takes a different pattern of reasoning. Think about having children and finishing a bachelor's degree. They may both be long-term goals, but some people have to choose which of those goals will be addressed first.

What would our society be like if it was mandated by law that everyone's first priority was to be a good person? What does *good* mean? I'm sure there would be just as many interpretations to that law as people it would govern. The point is that all of us have different priorities, and yet do you really take the time to sit down and write them down? Do it now.

List the top three priorities in your life.

1. _____

2. _____

3. _____

Was it hard? Did you write down the first three things that came to your mind? Most people would write family, health, and money. Does it surprise you that *peace of mind, good self esteem* or *living a thoughtful life* doesn't come to mind as quickly? There is nothing wrong with the first three things. These are what usually give us a sense of well-being. If you had to continue your list to **add three more things**, what would they be?

1. _____

2. _____

3. _____

It is usually when we have some priorities in our lives that we are the happiest. Oftentimes, *trust fund* kids feel empty and misguided because they don't have to worry about making money or obtaining things they thought would make them happy. Would these same individuals feel just as empty if they had the same financial pressures that most of us do? Maybe. Yet having a clear idea of what gives our life value and purpose can be rewarding and comforting. How did you feel about writing your priorities down? *(I had to ask: it's my training).*

Patients come in all the time and state what they want (their priorities) in coming to my office. They may decide that getting rid of the depression or being less anxious throughout their day is a priority. If an addiction is a problem, not having any stress or feelings may be a priority, yet the real priority is continuing in their addictive behavior.

Our priorities are not always in our best interest. You may need to stop and ask yourself if what you are setting up as your priority will really meet your needs.

There have been times in my life where I had to have the latest *toy* or the quickest deal on a car. It was only after the fact that I realized how off base my so-called priority was—yet it seemed so important at that moment.

One of the advantages of reading a book like this is to gain some insight into your choices earlier rather than later.

Here is an exercise in taking responsibility for your choices in life. **List at least five things you set as priorities and later realized that they weren't all that important**. *(You may want to keep a journal as you read this book: really get into the exercises and process your thoughts.)*

1. _____

2. _____

3. _____

4. _____

5. _____

Now think about (and write about) what you didn't do because the above 5 things were the priority.

_____

_____

_____

_____

There were times when I didn't spend time with someone I loved because I had to do something else instead. Regrets? Yes. When someone you loves dies suddenly, a common thought might be: "I would love to have one more chance to let him know _____." People's ideas may differ, but the take-home message is universally: "I wish I would have _____.
Hopefully those feelings of regret can be used to learn and set priorities more carefully.

Picture the scenario where you are coming home from work and you are tired. You really just want to sit down, have some quiet time and NOT BE BUGGED! If you could throw on a sweatshirt that says in large letters "LEAVE ME ALONE," you would do it in a heartbeat. Yet here come the kids yelling, or the dog, or your parents are expecting you for dinner in 30 minutes. You probably do not give yourself time to reason whether or not you will give any or all the above your time because they are priorities in your life. You just do it.

Would you feel the same if a long-lost friend called the minute you walked in the door and asked you to meet for a drink? You would probably state that you already had plans *(even if you didn't)*, and explain that if you had been given more notice, you would be there. Why the white lie? A spontaneous drink with your friend was not a priority at that moment.

How do you decide what your priorities are? Do you have a hard time doing this at work? You have probably had a routine that makes you comfortable. I know that my priority is to see my patients, then maybe return phone calls, then open mail and do bills, etc. It seems pretty clear.

If I try to make my time out of the office as simple, can I do it? I have learned to do it with the simple things: buy groceries, go to the bank or the cleaners, meet a friend, or go to a talk. I first check in with myself as to how I feel. *(If that wasn't your immediate thought, go back to the Chapter 1 and read it again.)* I then ask myself, "What is the worst case scenario if I don't make it to the store or the cleaners? Will I starve or have to go naked to work tomorrow?" NO. I have some choices. Am I tired? What do I want to set as my priority at that moment?

The choice I make may differ on any given day. I remember when I did not give myself the choices; it was like I had a drill sergeant in my head saying, "Do it." What were the consequences? I would finally get home, exhausted, forgetting two or three things I really wanted to get and be angry. I have since learned to *not sweat the small stuff.*

What about the *big stuff*? I just returned from a workshop where the therapist asked the audience if there was anyone who had a problem they couldn't solve.

A girl raised her hand, and her dilemma was that she was pregnant and wanted to stay home with her baby for at least the first twelve weeks. She was allowed only six weeks for maternity leave from her work, and she had to decide if she was going to jeopardize her job by staying out twelve weeks, or give up her desire to stay with her baby.

The therapist asked her to pick someone out of the audience to be the part of her that knew what was best for her. I was picked and sat facing her. She was asked to tell me what *her true self* was telling her around her decision. I was then supposed to echo back to her what she had said. *(It was a good thing I was listening!)* I told her that she had lost jobs before, always managed to find another one, and she had never let herself go hungry. She knew that she really wanted to bond with her baby.

The therapist then had her pick someone to be her *guardian angel* and listen to the response I was giving. The girl looked at me and started her *yes, but's* and *what if's*. The angel told her to trust herself and her beliefs.

It finally became clear that her real dilemma was not about the choice to work or not. She really had decided her baby was her priority. Her dilemma was her spirituality and lack of belief.

What does this example teach us? We really do know ourselves better than anyone, and when we take time to set priorities, we can think pretty clearly. We tend to get into trouble when we set them without thinking through the pros and cons. That is when the *if only's* set in.

List your top five priorities in your life.

1._____

2._____

3._____

4._____

5._____

Did you jot them down in a minute this time, or did you think about them and do the pros and cons? If you give it more time, did they change? Were they really yours or ones you thought you should put down?

I was obviously excited to write this book and am just sitting back down to finish this chapter. Why the interruption? It was time to pick up my father who is 90, eat together, and then play cards. Is finishing this book a priority. Sure! Is still having my dad around to play cards a bigger one? No contest.

We make choices, and we try to make them *good enough*. No, I didn't say *perfect* because that's a setup. I have never met a *perfect* human being. Have you?

If you have not listed yourself as a priority, then we have some more work to do. Are you expecting others to do it for you?

Our priorities change as we age. In our teens, our tasks are to develop social skills and learn about relationships *(as well as drive our folks nuts)*. If you are now a parent, can you think back to some of your behaviors as a teen? Did you set your parents' needs as a priority back then? I doubt it.

A few years ago, I looked at my folks and asked them when they had gotten smart again. Because at 16, I was convinced that they were both dumb; and not only did I let them know it, I told all my friends how dumb they were! It is funny how they regained their smarts! Go figure.

Most of us in our 50s who are fortunate enough to have parents still with us would probably list them now as one of our top priorities. When you think of your 20s, it was probably finding a mate, starting a family, and working in your career. In your 40s and 50s, your priorities change again to the grandkids, or hopefully helping others along their journey and re-defining your needs. I live with people in their 60s and 70s, and it's interesting to see that their health concerns become a priority—something that didn't even cross their minds in their 20s.

Hopefully by the time we reach our 40s and above, we have had some experience in setting our priorities. You've bought this book. Will it be a priority to finish it? What is it about your mental health that helped you decide to buy it? Is feeling good about yourself and your life a priority? *(I hope so!)*

If you often feel overwhelmed and have a challenging time completing what you have started, remember the following story that came from a Franklin training on time management:

"If we both were standing on the roof of the tallest building in the city and it was adjacent to another tall building, and I put a board between the two, would you walk the board for $10,000?"

(Most people laugh and say, "No way!")

"What if I tell you that it is sprinkling and the board is getting damp, but I will up the price to $50,000? Now will you walk across it?"

(Some people may hesitate, but most again give an emphatic "No!")

"Well, what if I tell you that now it is raining, but I will up the price to $100,000?"

(Most people still wouldn't risk their lives for $100,000.)

"If I had one of your children and threatened to throw them off the building if you didn't walk across, would you do it?"

(Most people don't even hesitate and say, "Of course!")

It is all about priorities and the way you set them. Understanding your priorities gives your life purpose. Then you can set your goals and make a commitment to meet them.

Chapter 4

Commitment to Work on
My Current Relationships and Roles

Oh, what a great gift we would have
if we could only see ourselves as others see us.
—Robert Burns, Scottish poet (1759-1796)

We all have roles in our lives. That is the healthy part. The part that
becomes unhealthy is when we get stuck in a certain role.

EXERCISE: Circle all the roles that apply to you:

Father	Mother	Child
Uncle	Aunt	Cousin
Grandfather	Grandmother	In-law
Husband	Wife	Godparent
Brother	Sister	Friend
Boyfriend	Girlfriend	Significant Other
Teacher	Colleague	Boss
Partner	Lawyer	Doctor
Executor	Accountant	Mechanic
Spiritual Advisor	Mentor	Housekeeper
Pet owner	Volunteer	

Job Title: _____

Other:_____

Can you see that it is starting to get complicated? I could continue
to list several more roles, but you get the idea.

Affirm:
I value my relationships
And work on honesty and appreciation to enrich them.

Now, list the relationships in your life that need improving.

_____

_____

_____

_____

Have you ever sat down and thought about how you could improve
these relationships? Most of my patients sort these on a *crisis basis*.
It is sort of like our health-care priorities. Do we spend as much
time on the routine visits and preventative tests as we do when we
are sick and feeling rotten? No. The same may go for our
relationships. We tend to focus on the ones that need it at the time
because of an argument or a need.

    Have you ever found yourself feeling responsible for an in-law?
This is a common complaint. "My husband (or my wife) expects
me to be the one to handle the surgery plans for _____
(talking about the mother-in-law or father-in-law)." When asked,
"What has kept your spouse from stepping up to the plate?" the
patient will look at me and say: "Well, it has always been this way;
it is assumed I will handle it!" Inquiring about the patient's
behavior, I ask, "What is it about you that you set yourself up as a
caretaker?"

    The consequences are feeling angry, resentful, and
unappreciated. Are they getting stuck in a role they really don't
want? Do they need to step back and look at their options? We may
spend a session on setting boundaries and letting them look at who
else might be available to meet the needs of the in-laws. Is there a
local country agency or eldercare group that can assist?

It is important to realize what roles you are taking on in life and ask yourself, "Is this really necessary, or is it causing more stress in my life?"

We all have roles in our lives, whether they be as son, dad, brother, accountant, coach, husband, etc. It is healthy to go back and forth in these roles. The problem starts when we get stuck in a role. If I were "THE DOCTOR" 24 hours a day, I would burn myself out and drive everyone around me crazy. I need to be able to shed my doctor role at the end of a day and slip into one of my other roles.

If you listed a relationship that needs improving, is it because you are *stuck* in that role, or is your partner? Can you imagine what I would be like as a friend, daughter, significant other, niece, dog-mom, or step-mom if I could not take myself out of the doctor role? Do you think that it would get old real quick? The starting point is to look at your degree of flexibility.

Recently I spent time with a friend who suffered a broken hip, and we had a great time catching up and just being together. It meant taking time off from the office and getting into my friend role. It was a quick decision because I knew I was needed, and my priority was to be with her. Did I get to the hospital and demand to see her X-rays? Did she ask me to run by radiology and take a look at her x-rays to give her my opinion? No, we both respected my role as her friend, not her doctor. She already had a doctor that was taking care of her hip. I was there to help her rally and feel supported.

Respect is so important in a relationship. Take a moment and ask yourself if any relationship on your *troubled list* is due to having difficulty with respecting one another.

If I asked you right now which relationship in your life needed a commitment of your time, which would you pick? When someone says to me, "You know me better than anyone," I think, "What a compliment!" I must have done something to establish a level of intimacy that is valued.

Where do you start to work on a relationship? We are back to the needs list.

- **What do you need from that person in the relationship?**

- **Is this the right person to meet my needs?**

A patient of mine was hurt and angry because she started using more of her pain patches than were prescribed, and her husband *did not say anything*.

I asked her why she thought this was so, and she responded that either he didn't care about her enough or that she had pulled "too much crap and he was fed up."

"Is there any possible other explanation for his behavior? Do you think it might be because he has *healthy boundaries*, and he knows that it is not his job to monitor your addictive behavior?"

She looked at me like I was crazy and said, "Come on, doc, he's my husband!"

"Exactly!" I told her, "and it is not *his stuff* to police your behavior. He is not your therapist or your psychiatrist or your recovery coach. A husband will lend you his car to go to a 12-step meeting, or call and make an appointment with your therapist if you are busy." I also told her to quit perpetrating him with her expectations and go to an NA meeting, to people who can meet her needs around helping her fight her opiate addiction. She was going to the wrong person to get her needs met and angry that it wasn't happening.

Then I added (as if she wasn't reeling enough), "Can you imagine going home and telling your husband that you need to make amends because you were expecting him to do something that was *your stuff*?"

She didn't know if she could do it without tears.

"So what?" Tears can be healing, and it's OK to be tearful.

I have to laugh when I remember walking through an airport with a good friend who had three older brothers and really grew up being doted on and taken care of by everyone in the family. We were nearing her gate when a woman said "Hi" to her and told her that she had better hurry up and get to the gate because the flight had been canceled, and everyone was trying to make other flight arrangements. She turned to me and said, "Do you believe that?"

I assured her that the fact that a flight was canceled was no big shocker to me.

She answered, "Do you believe that she didn't come with me to make sure I made it onto another flight?"

I looked at her and inquired if this was a close friend of hers. She assured me that she was an acquaintance and didn't see her much. I told her to wake up and smell the coffee. It wasn't that woman's *stuff* to make sure she was taken care of. There were airline personnel available she could go to for help. My friend definitely was setting herself up by expecting someone to *help her* that had given her a clear sign that she wasn't on the same wavelength. We later laughed about it (after we had both aged and she had been through therapy). She needed to recognize that she had to pick someone who was willing to meet her needs in order to avoid feeling rejected.

It never fails to amaze me that when I ask a patient what they want most in a relationship with another person, the first answer is usually **respect**, which is then followed by honesty. Yet, they expect their friend/significant other to know exactly what they mean by those terms. What looks like respectful behavior to one person may be totally different to another. How do you show others you respect them? Keep their confidences? Not call after 10:00 p.m.? Follow their advice? It may take different behaviors. So I ask them to fill in the following sentence:

Would you be willing to _____**?**

Several times, I will see responses like *hear me* or *be affectionate* or *pay attention to me*. One person's definition of those behaviors may be much different than their partners. Therefore, I will ask them to be specific and give behavioral guidelines such as: "Would you be willing to sit with me on a Monday and Thursday evenings from 9:00 to 9:20 p.m. and just listen? And not try to solve anything, criticize, or judge—just listen?" The more specific you can be in stating your needs, the less there is room for misinterpretation.

EXERCISE: Write down three behavioral guidelines for your friend/ parent/spouse/significant other and see if it helps you feel that your needs will be met.

1. _____

2. _____

3. _____

DO <u>NOT</u> ASK FOR THEM WHEN THE OTHER PERSON CAN'T LISTEN TO YOU, such as in the middle of an argument, or when s/he is soaking in a tub and needs quiet time. Set yourself up for success with good timing!

There is something about writing your needs down. You own them in a different way, and people can then read them and decide if they choose to meet them.

One of the exercises that my patients hate is to write down in a food journal everything they put in their mouths. The resulting grimace on their faces is indicative of how they perceive this activity as potentially painful.

"Is there another way to look at it?" Many patients claim that they resisted eating something because they didn't want to write it down. This exercise increases awareness and allows them to question their *needs* at the moment. When they truly commit to the exercise, they come in with a working document that is folded, torn, stained—not a neat computer-generated sheet done by memory. Some of them expect their significant other to be their food police. This is going to the wrong person to meet their need to decrease their food intake: it is their job!

Sometimes I ask couples or a parent and an adolescent to draw up a contract which states the behaviors that need to change and the consequences if they don't. If the commitment is to better a relationship with a teen, then a contract can work.

A teenage patient wanted to stay up on the weekends as late as he wanted. His parents complained that if they allowed it, the next day he would be crabby and wouldn't get his chores completed. I asked them to write a contract stating that he could stay up; but if he was moody or oppositional the next day, he lost the privilege the next weekend. They came back and stated that things were great. He was staying up, and the next day he was doing what he was expected to do in a pleasant mood.

It takes time to look at someone whose relationship you value and give that person the respect, kindness and attention s/he deserves. The *needs list* helps to stop the guessing and make the most out of time spent together.

By now, you probably realize that you have a lot of needs that require a lot of interactions with various people in your life. Have you thought about the various levels of intimacy that each of these people share with you? Would you go to your dry cleaner when you are upset and need a hug, or to the local bank teller or your mail person? I hope not.

You have spent time and energy developing different relationships with different people. Have you earned the right to ask for certain things? Have your efforts in the relationship been genuine?

Mary came in and during her evaluation stated that she had been married for 23 years and started to complain that her husband tuned her out and never seemed to be there for her emotionally. I asked her if she wanted to stay in the relationship, and she said that she did but was very unhappy. We started to explore her relationship, and she said that he really never was emotionally available, but she was busy with raising the kids and then went back to school. She now found that since the kids had moved out or no longer needed her as much, she was having more together time with her husband and feeling lonely. They had never been in couple's therapy since he seemed content in the relationship, and she felt she never had the time.

I asked her what she was willing to do to work on the relationship and she responded with, "I don't know." She was afraid to *rock the boat* but did agree to write down some of her *needs* in the relationship. It never dawned on her to really look at what she expected from him, or if it was her *stuff* around the kids leaving and struggling with her need for acceptance. She agreed to work on her issues in addition to her relationship issues.

A variety of answers come from asking couples that have been together for years, "What helped?"

"Never go to bed angry."

"Do unto others as you would have them do unto you."

"Pay attention to body language, facial expressions, and keep your sense of humor."

I had to laugh when I asked my father if there was anything he felt he wanted to know about my mother. (They had been married for 62 years.)

He looked at me and said, "If I don't know it by now, then I don't need to know it."

I guess there is a point when you can say, "Enough!" Yet the feeling that comes with watching people really enjoy and value one another is priceless. Did they always have that special connection? Rarely. It took work; but for those that did the work, they agree: it is the relationship that helps give their lives value. The commitment my folks made to each other 62 years ago held up in spite of some hard times.

Frequently I ask my patients what they need from me and how they see my role in their lives. If the answer includes a *fourth for bridge next weekend* or *instructions in applying for Medicare* or *help in choosing the right insurance company*, then I have to help them understand our relationship. A doctor-patient relationship has boundaries, and the agreement patients sign clarifies my expectations of their behavior. If they cannot respect those boundaries, they may be asked to find another doctor.

What happens when you get too needy? You tend to push people away. Some patients feel that in order to feel *worthy*, they have to go from crisis to crisis. If friends and family continually save them, then they feel someone cares. They really don't *get it* that the behavior sets them up to live in chaos and attract others who behave in a similar manner. People get burned out with that level of intensity.

Here is an exercise for you to evaluate if you are healthy in seeking support, or if you are possibly burning people out with neediness. Healthy relationships require balance: respect for your needs, and at the same time, respect for the roles others play in your life.

EXERCISE:

1. **Write down to whom you turn for *help*.**

2. **Identify how many times in the last month you have called on that person to meet one of your needs.**

3. **Are you being reasonable?**

4. **Is that his/her role?**

Name of person	# times/mo.	Reasonable?	His/her role?

Once you have identified the various roles you have in your life, the next step is to set and honor boundaries in these relationships.

Chapter 5

Commitment to Set Healthy Boundaries

**There's only one corner of the universe
You can be certain of improving,
And that's your own self.**
—Aldous Huxley, British novelist (1894-1963)

Let's say that you are worried about your partner who is having a problem with a substance, whether it is alcohol, food, marijuana, cocaine, sedatives or opiates. *(I already addressed an example of the man who wanted his wife to monitor his pain medication usage and was angry that she chose not to and keep her boundaries.)* You may need or want your partner to stop using, yet will quickly realize that if you continue to try to control that person's behavior, you'll just get more frustrated. The moment you use *you* statements rather than *I* statements, people tend to shut down because it sounds accusatory. "*You* need to stop" as opposed to "*I* am concerned about your use" is an example of how a subject may be approached. This way you are staying in your role as partner and not crossing the boundary into therapist.

I tell a patient's partner that they can't be the patient's therapist, psychiatrist or recovery coach; they need to stay in their role, whether it is wife, husband, spouse, or significant other. It is especially difficult for those who are co-dependent—those who are so busy taking care of other people's needs that they never feel that their needs are being met.

One of my patients is always jumping in to "save the underdog" (his definition), and this has led him to being beaten up, avoided, and angry to the point where it has affected his health. He had decided that a woman he worked with had been treated badly by her boyfriend. He decided to go over to their house (uninvited) and "straighten him out." Needless to say, the boyfriend didn't appreciate this, things escalated, and my patient was arrested. He now realizes after I have asked him at least two dozen times, "DID THEY ASK FOR YOUR HELP?" He **does** have a choice to either respect the boundaries of others or else continue to *react* with his *saving-the-underdog* behaviors. The goals in his therapy are to learn to step back, consider his options, and then *take action*. We came up with other behaviors he could have used if he was concerned for her well-being. Can you think of some alternatives?

Another frequent complaint that I hear is: "I don't understand why no one ever *appreciates what I'm trying to do!* I feel so alone and yet nothing I do seems to work." This person may walk into my office and say, "Doctor, I think I've been depressed all my life."

One of my teachers responded to this statement with:

I get it!
A depressed sperm hit a depressed egg,
and there you were!

They may go on to state, "Things never seem to be *good enough.*" (Did you catch the global words: *always, never,* and *nothing*?) It must be so hard to go through life convinced that things will never change. Next time you catch yourself using the words "I *always,*" consider it a red flag. Why haven't you changed your behavior if it has kept you in the problem?

A problem is that they look externally for a sense of well-being. It is difficult for them to find it inside themselves. We may start to look inward by defining what gives value to their lives. Is it their family members or their spiritual beliefs? They are so reactive to other people's thoughts, feelings, words, and actions that their boundaries with others are blurred. They will do practically anything to help solve someone else's problems.

Did my patient who decided to defend his female co-worker **care** about her? Sure. Was he a compassionate and caring person? Yes. My point in writing about boundaries is not to keep our distance from meeting other people's needs, but to understand that it is their (the other people's) job to identify their needs and then ask us for our help if they want us involved. Do you think the person who feels his actions aren't appreciated really checked in with the person? Did he commit to a healthy boundary by first asking if that person preferred to work it out herself?

Consider the 14-year-old girl who comes in and tells me she is angry that her step-mom went to the fair with her office pals instead of asking her father. She felt that her step-mom should have taken her dad since they had recently been married (even though she and her sister vetoed the marriage).

"How did you hear about her choice of going with her office pals?"

She said that she heard them arguing through the walls and that her dad told her all about it in the morning.

I then asked her: "Are you owning your dad's anger for him?"

She looked at me with a blank look and assured me that it was *her* anger.

I then suggested that maybe it was a matter that should stay between her step-mom and her dad. I really wanted to see what *her* anger was about. Right away I figured that her dad probably didn't have the greatest ability to set boundaries if he was discussing his feeling about his wife with her daughter and not keeping it between him and his wife.

Knowing how to set boundaries comes with knowing what is your *stuff* and what belongs to other people. We all have heard the phrase

TMI (too much information); and if this fits, it usually means that someone is overstepping boundaries and you are feeling uncomfortable. Did you ever ask yourself: "Why?" Maybe it is because when someone shares information with you, there is an unsaid expectation that now that you have the information, you'll do something.

I was working out in the gym when another acquaintance came in and said "Hi" and proceeded to tell me about his sexual relationship with his wife. I quickly waved my white towel, told him that I was *off duty,* and the topic was not appropriate gym conversation. Boundary violation? *(Well, ya think?)*

If you sometimes feel that you have that red target on your forehead that pulls people in to confide their problems, you might want to ask yourself if your boundaries are appropriate. A friend can listen and refer someone into counseling. A good response sometimes is to address the feelings: "You sound angry. Would you be willing to discuss that with a therapist?"

Too often we are drawn in and start to feel trapped or held hostage by someone else's feelings. Does this sound familiar? Try to remember that you can control only your thoughts, feelings, behaviors and actions—no one else's!

When you picked up this book, were you thinking that you needed some adjustment in your attitude, self esteem, and to focus on yourself? Or others? It may be that you feel overwhelmed with other people's *stuff.*

Some days, I get the point where I don't want to answer the phone, thinking it is someone who wants me to *do* something. Does that thinking serve me? If I'm feeling frustrated or overwhelmed, then it is my job to check in with myself and see if I have set the needed boundaries with people in my life.

When I covered another psychiatrist's practice, the patients came in and always asked: "Where's _____?"

It struck me that they referred to the psychiatrist by her first name instead of Dr. _____. I knew it was going to be a long week because the boundaries had not been set with her patients. I had fun watching them look surprised when they asked what they should call me, and I replied: "Dr. Berkus."

We then processed their feelings when I didn't offer my first name.

I felt that they needed a doctor, not a friend. Do I always insist on my title? No. It has more to do with the patients and what their needs are in the doctor–patient relationship.

Frequently, patients will ask me to "call in something" for their urinary tract infection or their birth control pills. I make it very clear to them that I will handle their psychiatric medications but not all their medication needs. Do they have a choice of whether to accept that or get angry? You betcha! *(I'm from Minnesota.)* If they get angry, I know right away that we have some boundary issues to discuss, and I could guess that they have difficulty with the *no* word.

If you are still unclear about the term boundary, watch a dog. They will let other dogs know pretty quickly what they feel is their territory. They have a very simple behavioral response to protecting their food, toys, or owners. I know in a heartbeat if I do something that infringes on my dog's space or things. We are still working to help him understand that he is not the ruler of everyone's universe, but he does think he is at the top of the pecking order.

I have a refrigerator magnet that states: "God help me to be the person my dog thinks I am." Think about it. I'm dependable because I take him out, feed him, play with him and really have no reason to betray, perpetrate, lie, cheat, take, abuse, get needy, or not meet his needs *(except when he pees in my closet, one foot from his doggy door)*. Of course he is going to think I am wonderful, and he shows it whenever I walk in the door: "Hiyahihahiyahiya."

In a lot of ways, the role of *doggy mom* is gratifying and easy. Where else would I get that kind of unconditional love? Other roles may be more complicated and demanding at times. It is up to me to find a way to get as much gratification from my other roles as I get from one so well defined as *dog mom*. I know it helps to be as open and direct with the others in my life and to be accepting of their *less-than-doggy* traits.

There have to be boundaries in healthy relationships. When I hear someone say, "I just love him or her to death," I cringe. *(Did they really kill their partner with love?)* I will consider how well each person in the relationship really listens, and when one person tends to answer for the other, I know we have a problem. I can watch families in the waiting room and tell by their behavior how the boundaries are set in the family. Kids complain all the time about how *mean* their parents are, and they just want to be left alone. I watch for triangulation. Does the mom ask the child to tell dad something, or does the child ask mom to ask dad? There is so much more room for misinterpretation when we create triangles instead of dyads (one-to-one communication).

So, how do you learn to set boundaries if you have never set them before? Slowly.

One of my patients pretty much does *everything* for her husband but gets very few of her needs met. She also lets her kids know that she is there whenever they need something. She will run herself ragged meeting their needs and then wonder why she is angry.

The first thing she needed to realize was that she wasn't going to *change* anyone else's behavior. Her family was now *trained* to expect her to meet their needs, and she wasn't going to be met with a lot of "go mom" when she changed the rules to meet her own needs.

Are there consequences for committing to healthier behaviors? Sure. I knew she was going to have a hard time (people pleaser that she was) to putting her own mental fitness first.

I had her make a list of things she had been putting off in order to take care of her family. Her assignment was to first let anyone who asked her to do something know that she would "think about it and get back to them." This would teach her to check in with herself and see what her feelings were about the request. If she decides that she doesn't want to run into town to pick up a prescription for her husband (which he could do himself), could she offer to do it the next time she is out near the pharmacy when it wouldn't mean a special trip? The boundary would be: "I would be happy to get it next time I'm out, but I'm not going to stop _____(whatever she was in the middle of) and go now. Would you be willing to either give me a little bit more notice or go get it yourself?" Now, he has the choice of honoring her decision or getting angry.

Most of us have learned some healthy boundaries such as not entering a bedroom or bathroom without knocking and asking permission, or not reading someone else's mail. We step back when people are keying in their pin numbers at an ATM to give them their privacy and space.

This chapter is about looking at others and understanding when it is appropriate to assist them and when it may be more beneficial to let them learn to problem-solve on their own. It can never hurt to check out your intentions with the person you want to help, and be gracious if they decide they don't need your help. Is this a novel idea for some of you?

If you are panicking because you are realizing that you may not be great at setting boundaries, RELAX. Compare it to people who have never learned to swim. Does that mean that they are good or bad? NO! It just means that they have not had the experiences like jumping into a pool and enjoying the coolness or the ability to float. I can try to explain to them how it feels to do somersaults or play Marco Polo, and they can imagine it, but it is not the same experience.

Can someone learn to swim as an adult? Yes, it is harder because of more fears, but it is manageable. Would I start by throwing someone into the deep end? Of course not. First, I would help them put their face in the water, then hang on to the side and learn to kick, then go to a paddleboard, etc.

There are steps to learning, and the same thing holds true for learning to set boundaries.

Now that you have an idea about boundaries, how many of your friends and family have good boundaries? Who does and who does not? How are you going to commit to model healthy boundaries for people around you?

Chapter 6

Commitment to Grow Spiritually

**One person with a belief
is equal to a force
of ninety-nine who have only interests.**
—John Stuart Mill, British philosopher (1806-1873)

We've all heard the stories of the mom who sees her child trapped under a car and somehow finds the strength to lift the car in order to save her child. We watched in amazement as a model clung to a tree for hours in incredible pain during the tsunami to survive and the man who was found buried for days yet hung on. The opposite is also true: we have seen seniors *lose their will to live* after the loss of a spouse.

How hard would each of us fight under similar circumstances? I was in tears hearing a wonderful man in a wheelchair state how grateful he was that his neck fracture was a centimeter lower than his friend's. Why? Because he still had the ability to bend his wrist and support his hand in an upright position. He challenged us: "Did you ever realize how important it is to be able to pick your nose?" His humor was so contagious that whenever I drop into a victim role, I hold my hand up and flex it at the wrist—a great reminder that my issues maybe aren't so big. Did he have a choice of how to respond to his physical challenges? We all have choices.

When evaluating a patient, I frequently ask if they are a *spiritual person*. I've gotten several interesting looks and answers. Most people explain to me that they either do or don't go to church or synagogue, or that they consider themselves *spiritual* but are not involved in an organized form of religion. Others tell me whether or not they have a belief in a higher power or whether they are tied into nature but don't believe that there is a higher power.

The purpose of this line of questioning is to help people decide what gives value and purpose to their lives. If they are coming to a psychiatrist, chances are they are in the middle of a crisis, or their mood has altered to the point that their depression, anxiety, or their ability to *feel good* is affected.

If people answer, "I seemed to have lost my spiritual connection" or "I'm not where I want to be in relation to my faith," we will start to explore the presence or absence of ritual in their lives. A colleague once told me not to ask about the willingness of patients to develop a morning ritual if I was not willing to keep one myself.

In the first chapter, I talked about the **Daily Psychological Inventory**, which was a way to check in with ourselves. This is different. The idea of starting a day with some sort of ritual is about centering yourself for the day to come. Several religions have a morning-prayer sequence or a process of becoming one with their surroundings. People who meditate or do some sort of yoga, tai chi or *time out* describe having a sense of inner peace.

By watching patients as they enter my office, I can learn a lot by how they approach a new environment. If they scan the room and let themselves take in the atmosphere, areas of comfort, options for self-soothing (there are dog books and a sand garden in plain view), it tells me something about their process. If they arrive out of breath (they didn't notice the elevator across from my office), late, anxious, and waiting to be directed, that indicates a different type of self-care. It has nothing to do with intellect or level of *dis-ease*. It tells me how they look inward to help themselves deal with a new or stressful situation.

How many times have you had someone stop walking right I front of you (no brake lights) as you were in a small area, such as departing a flight or at the top of an escalator? Are they thoughtless, stupid, inconsiderate, or just lost in their thoughts, their space, and their needs? Next time you experience this, use it to take notice of your position in regards to others. Are you being mindful?

A better example of mindfulness may be by describing how some travelers handled their transport from the airport to a wonderful resort in the mountains. *(I just happened to catch a ride since I knew the driver.)* It was a beautiful day and the clouds were forming a shade pattern on the mountains. The sun was also starting to set, and the setting was extraordinary. Yet the visitors were oblivious to the scenery around them. They were complaining about the trip and the flight delay. I kept waiting for one of them to pause and comment on their new environment as we were on a back road in the country. It never happened, and instead I heard a lot of questions about what was available for them to do at the resort and how their time was scheduled.

I struggled to keep my mouth shut *(good boundaries—I wasn't their psychiatrist or therapist)* because I really wanted to yell: "Hey, are you blind? How can you not appreciate what is in front of you!" *(Not too perpetrating, huh?)* Evidently, my *stuff* was big at the moment. Yet I felt like all I was hearing was the "big I" from each of them: *I want. I need. I hope. I can't wait.*

Sometimes it is hard to acknowledge that there are more than our needs at any given moment. I hope that the awareness starts that several other people with the same thoughts surround us. Does it serve us in the long run? Can you see how their trip might have had a special gift if they had noticed what was around them?

This is a fairly typical example of how we drift from **a sense of being in the moment**.

The spirituality I'm referring to is more of an awareness of where we are at any given moment, not just the times we turn to a higher power for guidance, support, comfort and relief. People may find their spirituality in religion or in their human experiences.

I spent five years in a Ph.D. program in Biochemistry. When in my first few months, sitting in a lecture given by a guest speaker, I was having trouble following the topic when one of the senior graduate students raised his hand and asked about the way a certain cellular mechanism may be working. I was clueless, and I remember thinking to myself, "How in the _____ did he come up with that?"

It was not until four or five years into my degree that I was the one in the front asking the questions that hopefully did not occur in everyone's mind. The point is that I had evolved in my level of thinking based on what I had learned about the body and how it works. I compare it to being told that you know when you are getting the hang of a foreign language when you can think and dream in that language.

**I feel that there is
a language of spirituality.**

**It starts
with an awareness of your position
and how you see yourself
with the things around you.**

We are exposed to so much sensory information in a day; there are reasons why we let a lot of information pass by.

AN AWARENESS EXERCISE:

• Close your eyes.

• If you are alone, try to describe the room you are in as if to a person who is sightless.

• If you are out and about, can you describe what the last two people you saw were wearing? How much can you recall?

• Do you remember the way you felt when you woke up this morning? What was your first thought?

• Think about the one person you have lost that causes that deep ache inside you. Can you…

    • Picture his or her smile?

    • Smell his cologne or her perfume?

    • Remember your last hug?

- As you think about this, are you smiling? Sad? OK with your thoughts?

There is an essence about that person that stays—whatever you what to call it—and that is the part of you that may help you examine your spirituality. It is a set of beliefs, experiences and personal inventory that makes you unique. Have you discovered yours?

This commitment to grow spiritually is sometimes the most difficult for people. This doesn't necessarily have to be about whether or not someone follows an organized religion.

> One of my patients had a theory. She thought that for the first year after the death of a loved one, the deceased could send some sort of signal to those left behind. It might look like a butterfly landing on them or lights left on in that person's room when no one was home to turn them on. Her favorite was a song (that would have meaning to the loved one) would come on when the person was thinking of the deceased.

Did this belief bring her comfort? Definitely. It was more of a feeling she would get than anything concrete. It gave her a sense of well-being that was valuable to her. The spiritual part of us can lead to a sense of something that gives us value and comfort as human beings.

Sometimes I long for the days when I had no idea why people behaved the way they do. That wonderful innocence I had as an undergraduate when I just looked but really did not see people the way I do now. I pick up intonations, behaviors, and reactions in an almost overwhelming manner on a daily basis, whether I'm waiting in line at the grocery store or watching people while sitting in an airport. Sometimes I want to shut myself off and just be.

I now do the same thing for me—AAAAH! I find myself watching my behaviors, thoughts, and actions, not in a paranoid way but rather as an observer of myself. It has just become second nature. I appreciate achieving this ability to live and focus on those things that *count* and give my life value instead of being caught up in the daily struggles and annoyances that seem to bombard us if we let them.

Right now, I am smiling because I am writing this on a plane while a sixteen-month-old is yelling and playing in the aisle. I remember a time when I would be muttering to myself: "That is why they make bulkheads, and my luck is to be stuck in this situation!" Now I watch his joy at his own voice and his discovery at each thing to grab in the seat. I am glad I can look at his essence or being and enjoy him instead of counting the minutes until we land and I am away from him. It is only a brief moment and experience in my life, yet it is impacting me. It is an experience to watch my own reactions and thoughts and recognize my own personal spiritual growth.

Awareness? Is the constant self-questioning and making choices a part of my spirituality and wonder at my world, or is it my own neurosis? It has saved me a lot of anger and frustration and has brought an appreciation of a force greater than mine that is somehow directing my abilities and experiences. Is it just brain chemistry? Is it something deeper?

Enough of the philosophy—I am just challenging each of you to look at the level you function with your thoughts and your actions. Is it where you want to be? Are you overwhelmed?

OK, let's say you want to start some sort of process of change.

Start with promising yourself to be in the moment.

If you can't do that, go back and watch your favorite animal or baby. Let yourself define where you are right now.

What brings you a sense of well-being? *(I am not talking about taking out your checkbook or pulling out pictures of the grandkids).* I am talking about taking a moment to see if you can *settle* and be OK with yourself right now. It is that ability that makes us different as humans. We have the ability to give this thought now. What comes into your mind? Can you speak to your higher power or check in with yourself without judging, commenting, or rushing? Just be.

Are you starting to get what I mean about a sense of self? If it is hard, it is OK to get help—whether it is with a cleric, teacher, friend, or other people you feel have achieved a level of their own spirituality that seems to make sense to you. Use your knowledge of yourself to decide what serves you and what does not. Be honest. Are you at peace with yourself, or do you need to work on it?

Chapter 7

Commitment to
Identify My Mind-Body Connection

**The very problem of mind and body suggests division;
I do not know of anything so disastrously affected
by the habit of division as this particular theme.**
—John Dewey

Did you ever find yourself *feeling bad* before an exam or a trip that you were not thrilled about in the first place? At a conference on fatigue and the effects of sleeplessness on the body, I was surprised to hear the following:

> **We each need about 8 (eight!) hours of sleep
> each night,
> and if we don't get it,
> we start to store up a *sleep debt*.**

The results of not listening to our body, and resisting the sleep it needs, can lead to a decrease in the body's immune system. It is amazing when people come into my office carrying a bag full of vitamins and supplements; yet when asked about sleep, they assure me that they can do just fine on four to five hours a night. Wrong!

The mind starts to shut down with lack of sleep *(ask any nurse or resident who has pulled call and were still expected to function).* The data is frightening on how little we perceive our own deficits.

How many of you have gotten behind the wheel of a car and convinced yourself that you were *OK to drive*? How about that incidence of jerking awake just in time to avoid an accident?

Before I went to medical school, my family practitioner told me that if I could convince my patients to give up cigarettes, eat healthy and wear their seat belts, I would be doing more good than by using anything I learned in medical school. *(So why did I put myself through all that?)* Naturally I didn't get it at the time. Now I realize that he was right, and if I could add getting the proper amount of sleep to the list, I would see far fewer patients.

Many of my patients complain of depression, which when we examine what they mean by that term, are really talking about fatigue, inability to sleep, and low energy. Some changes in their ability to fall and stay asleep may be all they need—not an antidepressant.

So why is sleep so low a priority for so many? We're too busy!!

List the five things you would do if you had an extra hour in every day.

1._____

2._____

3._____

4._____

5._____

It didn't take you long, did it? The point is that we are constantly pushing ourselves when the thing our bodies need most is to sleep. The "I'll just rest and sit still for ten minutes and be good as new" doesn't cut it.

You need to sleep!

When was the last time you took an inventory of the basic things you can do for yourself in order to allow your mind to function? Since I work with patients who tend to restrict their food intake, I basically tell them that in order to function, their brain has to marinate in good stuff *(medical term)*. Do you find yourself getting irritable when you are hungry?

People in recovery use an acronym **HALT**, meaning do not let yourself get too

Hungry
Angry
Lonely, or
Tired.

The chance of relapsing (whether it is drinking, gambling, eating, sexually acting out, reacting in a way you wish you hadn't, etc.) is greater when you are vulnerable to one on these states.

We also tend to make poor choices in terms of our general behavior when we have *checked out* and are not aware of our physical state. So how do you know if you get enough sleep? It would be great if I could order a blood test to give you that answer, but I can't.

The closest thing to an answer would be to have a week off and sleep as much as you wanted *(pay off time for your sleep debt)*, and then look at what you can accomplish and how you are functioning. If your level of functioning is much higher (better concentration, memory, and focus), then you have your answer.

How can you start to take care of yourself? **Power naps are great**—naps that are less than 45 minutes so that you don't let yourself go into REM sleep which is the stage of sleep where you dream and your body (except for diaphragm and eyes) is paralyzed. If you have ever been awakened from a sound dream and can't move, it can be frightening but will end as you become more aroused. During this time the body is rejuvenating, and you normally increase your REM sleep in the early morning; so setting the alarm early to *get an early start* is <u>not</u> in your best interest. You'll be feeling more tired.

You have probably heard the expression *good-sleep hygiene*. This really means trying to **commit to** a routine at night, whether it is soft music, a warm bath, or reading things that will not increase your blood pressure *(don't work on your tax return)*. If my patients are staying up late, I will ask them to start backing their bedtime by 30 minutes at a time: if they are going to bed at midnight, I will ask them to back it up to 11:30 p.m. and keep doing that every week until they have a more reasonable number of hours per night of quality sleep. Keeping a consistent bedtime and awakening time will optimize your sleep. Patients frequently smile when I suggest that the bed be used only for sleep or sex—not watching television, reading, or eating. The idea is to train your brain that a horizontal position means sleep. The body will adapt, and as your sleep normalizes, you will feel better.

The most striking mind-body connections I have seen are in psychiatric conditions where a patient may feel they are having seizures, but it is more of a stress response (pseudo-seizure) than a neurologically based disorder. This is also seen in conversion disorders.

> When I was doing my residency, I was on my neurology rotation (dealing with the nervous system: brain, spinal cord, strokes, and seizures) when I was called by the psychiatry resident to "come over to their ward to see a patient who knew me." I walked into the ward, and the attending physician *(top of the food chain)* told me he had ordered a CT scan because this patient couldn't move his arm and had asked for me by name.
>
> I walked into the patient's room, and he looked at me and started waving his *paralyzed arm* at me and said, "You're never home and you never answer your phone!"
>
> The hair on the back of my neck was standing up as the attending physician and the resident were staring at me. All I could think to say was: "I think you can cancel the CT scan."

It turned out that I had treated this patient on the neurology service when he had overdosed on his lithium (a medication used to treat mood swings). I had spent time with him in the ICU and had met his family. I didn't know what an impression I had made since it had been a year since I had seen him. I changed to an unlisted number, but the point is that he really believed that his arm was paralyzed and could not feel the pin pricks or tests the doctors used to initiate a response. This is an example of an extreme mind-body connection and is called a conversion reaction.

I'm not insinuating that we get to that level of impairment *(it is relatively rare)*, but it does follow that when patients start watching their choices of food (notice I didn't say *diet*: consider the first three letters of that word) and exercising, their body *gives back* and they feel stronger. Some people actually get psychotic (hallucinate or experience paranoia) by using too much caffeine.

It always amazes me when I do trauma work because people are so resilient. There have been patients who have experienced severe physical trauma, and they have no memories of their accident: their minds seemed to shut down, probably a protective mechanism. I laugh when I hear that from mothers who are pregnant with their second child and they describe the birth of their first child as *not that bad.* Maybe another type of protective mechanism?

The idea of hunger and craving is another example of the mind-body connection. A colleague uses this example: if you were hungry and your brain was sending signals for you to eat, you would be happy to be offered Brussels sprouts to extinguish the hunger. If you decided that you would pass on the offer, then it is not about hunger—it is about cravings. I have worked with people who "don't let themselves experience hunger." They have gotten into the habit of eating so frequently that hunger is not a normal cue for them. Then there are those who binge eat and eat right through the feeling of being full.

Our bodies will adapt to these behaviors by decreasing the signals normally sent. One example of this came from having people with anorexia swallow pressure balloons. It was determined that most people's stomachs will relax prior to a meal in readiness to receiving food. This was not the case in patients who has restricted their food intake and had a high level of fear around eating. Their stomachs remained rigid.

The advertisement industry knows how to affect our thinking. The television or movie screens flashing pictures of popcorn and candy stimulate us to raid the refrigerator or pantry, or to hit the snack counter, even if we had not considered it earlier. Our sense of smell and sight work to start us salivating and craving things we normally would not think about.

Ever go crazy in an airport and buy stuff you would never eat at home? I have sat waiting for a plane and watched people walk by with ice cream, large pretzels, and other fast food; and it seems many people *lose all rational thought* as they impulsively hit the fast-food counters. Is it a response to feeling no control on whether their plane is on time, or the fact that so many others are in control of their life until the trip is over? What happens to your commitment to eat healthy when you see all the foods that are available? It is almost like a mass hysteria: "Why am I eating a cinnamon roll when I would never do that at home?"

The take home message is that a healthy body and a healthy mind go together. If we listen to our body signals and take care of ourselves, the payoff would be great. So, put it back in perspective.

> If I offered each of you one million dollars to commit for the next week to eating healthy, getting eight to ten hours of sleep per night, reducing your stress levels with exercise, and making sure that the people you are involved with really have your best interest at heart, would you do it?

Priorities again.

The number of patients who complain of stomach upset, constipation, muscle aches, shortness of breath, and heart palpitations usually have had the medical work-up to determine the cause of these symptoms. This is appropriate and should be completed. It is after the work-up that the primary care physicians, internist, gastroenterologist, and gynecologist send their patients to a psychiatrist.

When I was a medical student working the family practice clinics, I thought that if I could have more time with each patient to address their psycho-social issues, I would be able to do more for the patient than just continue their pain medications for chronic back pain, regulate their insulin, and give medications for gastric reflux and sleep. Many patients were dealing with stressors that explained their headaches, lack of sleep, panic, anxiety, and depression.

Medications are useful as an effective *bridge* to get a person through the most difficult parts, decrease the symptoms, and give them an opportunity to more easily take care of themselves in more natural ways. Here is Angie's story:

> "I just hate my body!" Angie looked at me with tears in her eyes. She came in with depression, and we worked to understand her fatigue and lack of appetite. She was devastated from having had a miscarriage three months prior. She lost twenty pounds and had dropped out of school because she could not concentrate. This was her first episode of depression, and she was reluctant to try medications.
>
> I tried to explain some of the hormonal changes that her body had been through in the last months as well as the effects of the rapid weight loss. I told her that the medications would help restore the normal chemistry of her brain, not add anything foreign to it.
>
> She listened as I explained what chemical changes occur with trauma and poor nutrition. She was able to agree to try a medication until she could feel *good enough* to start eating again and focus on thoughts other than her loss. I was pretty confident that her fatigue, loss of appetite, weight loss, and lack of exercise were tied into her depression.

What do you do if you just lost your job and the rent is due, your child had to be rushed into the hospital after a head injury, or you've just been diagnosed with a breast lump and it needs a biopsy?

**No one prepares us to deal with crisis situations,
so the body reacts to the stress.**

When you have had traumas in your life, what physical complaints do you usually get at these most stressful times? In designing a program for stress reduction, which of these options would yours include? Biofeedback? Acupuncture? Massage? Exercise? Meditation? Reading? Time for fun? What else?

_____

_____

_____

Children will be brought in because they don't want to go to school or they have had numerous physical ailments. They may tell their moms that they have a tummy ache, or they "just don't feel good." They do not have the level of ability to abstractly put it together that the fear, loneliness, and sadness they are feeling may be adding to their pain. We work with the family to understand what has been going on in their lives and try to teach the kids how to deal with the situation.

Children will often follow their parent's cues. If they hear that mom has too much going on and it has given her a headache, they then start to form similar behaviors. Some people were raised to *be good* because one of the parents had a chronic illness or an anxiety disorder. In their minds, they could make it worse by misbehaving, so their world became one of avoiding stressors so they can keep someone *healthy and happy*. The behavior of being hypervigilant can lead to all sorts of physical ailments.

Are you aware of your *weak* areas in terms of health? Are you a stomach reactor or someone who is prone to headaches when stressed? What are you doing to keep your stress level under control? Are you on medications? If so, list the one(s) you are taking.

_____

_____

- If applicable, how many of them do you feel are due to stress-related symptoms? Which symptoms?

  _____

  _____

- How about seeing the proverbial glass as half full instead of half empty? What is an example of how you could do this?

  _____

  _____

- Are you in a *victim role* feeling trapped in some way in your life? If so, how?_____

  _____

  _____

- Are you constantly tired or lonely? _____

- What new behavior(s) will you to commit to so that you can decrease your stress? _____

  _____

  _____

  _____

Remember this book is about increasing your awareness and changing. Commit to understanding the link between your mind and body to empower yourself to be more mentally fit.

Chapter 8

Commitment to Change My Self-Talk

**Self-knowledge and self-improvement
are very difficult for most people.
It usually needs great courage
and long struggle.**
—Abraham Maslow, American psychologist (1908-1970)

The idea of being amused by yourself or considerate of your needs takes practice. Babies left alone giggle and explore their toes and fingers, and it seems so simple. The commitment to become aware of our self-talk can be so enlightening.

I have had the pleasure of meeting some Olympic athletes who have shared their stories of how they succeeded to such a high standard of performance. They acknowledged that they needed their coaches in order to help them maintain their focus and determination. The idea of getting up every day to run regardless of the weather, status of their health, degree of fatigue or of motivation: they would do it because they had made a commitment to their coaches. They learned to remind themselves of their priorities on a daily basis and go on to great successes.

"What is the one thing that bugs you the most about the way you're feeling?"

Joe responded, "I can't stop going over and over in my head everything I said when I'm in a social situation. I critique myself and usually wind up calling myself stupid, but I can't stop. I continually ask myself why didn't I say this or stand up for that. It seems so easy for everyone else. I feel awkward and foolish and am not surprised I don't have a lot of friends. I've been staying away when the few friends I have invite me out. I'm such a loser!"

Joe was setting himself up as his own judge and jury and finding himself guilty over and over again. His constant negative self-talk and self-hatred was keeping him isolated and alone. He found it uncomfortable if someone tried to pay him a compliment and told himself, "They were just being nice."

We started his process by trying to understand what he felt he did that warranted that level of verbal self-abuse. He eventually started to realize that it was his fear of rejection that kept him doing the rejection first—before anyone else could. He knew that it didn't feel good, but at least it was comfortable in it's predictability. He admitted that he was afraid to let me know what these conversations sounded like, but he knew he had to take the risk in order to get better.

• How many times do you find yourself listening to the *judge*?

• Does it seem like s/he is perched up on your shoulder and is chattering away at you?

• Do you have messages of "you're too fat, lazy, slow, stupid, ugly, repulsive, etc." that play over and over in your mind like a tape recorder stuck on one track?

• Do you give review your performance or the words that come out of your mouth constantly?

Most of us know when we are in the wrong—that is not what I am talking about. It is the *stinking thinking (a recovery term)* that keeps people stuck in their behaviors. When people are convinced that they don't deserve to be loved, or that no one could ever find them attractive, it will play out in their actions. They may avoid eye contact, or put themselves down before someone else can do it. Some people use sarcasm or humor to keep others at arm's length rather than risk letting someone get to know them. Others may behave in a way (start fights, be critical) that will push people away before they can be rejected. It doesn't feel good, but at least the outcome is predictable.

Take a moment and **list three messages that you give yourself that you would like to get rid of for good.**

1._____

2._____

3._____

You ask, "Now what?" Let's examine some options.

EXERCISE: Reverse the Thought

Step One: Pretend that just for today you will reverse the thought.

Step Two: Identify the negative thought.
     Maybe you have messages similar to some of these: "I never get a break." "I will never be thin." "I will die in this job before I try something else." "I am a bad person."

Step Three: Create an opposite message for yourself.
     So the "I am a bad person" becomes "I am a good person." You may play with the message, "I just may explore finding a new job" to replace "I will die in this job before I try something else."

Step Four: Think of an action you could take to act on that thought.
     If your thought changed from "I'm a bad person" to "I'm a good person," the action might be to do a favor for a friend or take

time to write down a list of your attributes. You may go on the Internet and explore a local charity that needs volunteers. See how it feels to commit to a different belief system about you. In recovery, there is a saying, *fake it until you make it*. Will it be easy to think of yourself in a different way? No!! Yet if you commit to making it a new habit, it will start to feel more comfortable.

Plenty of my patients seem to get stuck in the "I can't ask for help" stage. They have either decided that if they do ask for help, they will be thought of as weak, or they will be taken advantage of by the person they are taking the risk of approaching. The biggest fear is rejection and may see a rejection of their request as a rejection of them. If you are wondering how to deal with this, go back and read the first few chapters on getting needs met. They may have received the "pull yourself up by the bootstraps" lecture when they were kids or received the message that it "wasn't acceptable to ask for help."

This is the kind of message that, as an adult, you can commit to changing to a more positive message.

Step Five: Observe how your feelings change.

Do your feelings go from anger or sadness to something more positive? We cannot hold two contradictory thoughts at once ("I'm a bad person" and "I'm a good person"). Remember, it will feel uncomfortable because it is a different way of approaching a long-standing negative thought. If it was too easy, then you need to go back and pick a message that you've been stuck in for a long time that hasn't served you. It takes time to practice new self-talk patterns.

When we have negative self-talk, it may play out in physical symptoms. You may experience headaches, an upset stomach, or muscle tension in your neck and shoulders. *(Think about what you read in the last chapter.)*

A therapist I know told me about an assignment that you may consider a stretch. **Look yourself in the mirror and say "I love you" several times a day.** Think about it: how many times do you tell yourself you *hate yourself*? Why is that so much easier? If telling yourself that you love yourself sounds too *over the top*, then start slower.

You could start with a **daily commitment to a more positive thought** such as "I will not allow myself to verbally put myself down today" or "I am OK." My personal favorite is the *good enough* principle. "I am *good enough*" is a way of saying, "I don't have to be perfect." I'll bet that you would never talk to a stranger, your boss, or a friend the same way you talk to yourself. Why the need to be so hard on yourself?

Another way to approach changing your negative self-talk is to **examine the origin** of some of your messages. Was this an old tape from your childhood? Did someone tell you that you would never amount to anything? You would be lucky to find someone decent to care about you? Remember, as a child, we don't have the ability to question these statements: we just accept them.

Now, you are an adult. We are back to the re-deciding part. You don't have to continue *their truths* or *untruths* as it may be. It is time to tell yourself that you can **make new beliefs** and **learn to act on them**.

I am always curious when patients come in and tell me that the rest of their siblings turned to drugs or alcohol, yet they managed to survive and make something of themselves. What did they tell themselves? How did they make it happen? They obviously were able to *erase* their previous tapes and stay in healthier self-talk to succeed. Those who can't let go of the negative things they heard growing up sometimes fall into the *victim* role.

The role of *victim* quickly becomes apparent when someone blames his or her lack of achievement on something or someone else. "I had to drop out of school to help support the family" or "the boss had it in for me from the beginning" are examples of people using external perceptions as excuses. The "it's not my fault" gets old when it comes to making changes. It gets as old as "it's *always* been this way." My response to "it's *always* been that way" is "*that is no reason to avoid change.*"

Why is it so difficult for some people to make the commitment to change and others see it as a challenge? I think it is because we either decide it's just too overwhelming or we get *comfortable enough* with taking risks.

Is it scary to think about taking risks? Sure! I would rather have a patient cry or get angry than one that *gives up*. Anger is a great tool to use in committing to make changes. We see this every day in people who continue to work for important causes, so what about committing to making yourself the *important cause*?

What makes it easy to continue negative messages? It may go back to the times when you are most vulnerable. (Remember **HALT**—**H**ungry, **A**ngry, **L**onely and **T**ired.)

Are you feeling a loss of control? The scale shows a weight gain, or you can't fit into a favorite pair of jeans? Did you burn dinner, not hear from someone you hoped would call, or get turned down for a promotion or a job?

Well, that is part of life, so what is it about that moment that you chose to turn the anger inward? Why is it so hard to remember all the things that are going right in your life when that moment hits? Can you stop and say to yourself, "OK, I hate hearing this, but yesterday the same person said this and I was really pumped." Maybe the next day a great job offer will replace the job you didn't get.

It is an ability to hang on to the good things when you hear something you wish you did not have to hear. Picture this ability to *see the big picture* as the opposite of black/white thinking. Remember you now know how to *take action* instead of *react*.

Some of us have less ability than others to hold onto good thoughts when we perceive something *bad* is happening. Do you know those people who seem to take things in stride most of the time? How do they do that?

It is about giving yourself more positive messages than negative. Isn't it remarkable how easy it is for the *judge* or the *critic* to pop up rather than our own *nurturing parent*?

What do I mean by *nurturing parent*? Most of us remember running to mom or dad when we were hurt or frightened for reassurance or comforting. How often do you do that for yourself? Do you tend to tell yourself: "It's OK: You'll get through this." or "You deserve to let it go?"

Write down the last thing that you needed nurturing for. (Let yourself feel like a child.)

Did you ask to be nurtured? Who did you go to? Did you go to some negative self-talk? Some people never have had a nurturing role model. I frequently hear things like: "My mom never told me she loved me" or "I never received a hug from my parents." I will ask them if there was someone in their life who provided some nurturing: a teacher, grandparent, neighbor, or a friend's mom. We have to start at the beginning if the answer is "no." They may have to realize that their caregiver may have been *stuck* in what we call a certain ego state.

We all have **three ego states** that we jump back and forth from: *a computer, a child,* and *an adult state*.

Let's say your significant other walks in the door at dinnertime and announces: "I'm pooped. I just want to lay down." You have a choice of how to respond.

- If you are coming from your *computer*, you might say: "I'm pooped too. Let's order in for dinner."

- If your *angry kid* pops up, you might respond: "I hate it when you expect me to take care of dinner! I worked today, too!" *(Can you see where this will lead?)*

- The final choice is the adult who, if in the *nurturing adult*, might say: "You look tired. Go lay down, and I'll make dinner."

- This is in contrast to the *punitive adult* who may say: "You always use that as an excuse to get out of making dinner." *(Notice the global judgmental in that statement?)*

The problems begin in a relationship when two people get stuck in their roles. Can you imagine *the computer* married to the *angry kid* or the *punitive parent* married to the *angry child*? What a recipe for disaster!

Now that you are aware of the choices you have, are you willing to look at your own behavior for the next 24 hours and see if you are *stuck* in one of these state, or do you give yourself options? Does anyone suggest that you might be judgmental *(punitive parent)* or that you never show your feelings *(computer)*? Think about it. It might fit.

If you are serious about making the commitment to change the self-talk going on, try out the ***nurturing parent*** for yourself. See if it can become automatic and replace the negative thinking that seems to come so easily.

If the negative self-talk has led to you physically hurting yourself such as hitting yourself or cutting on yourself, then that is a signal that help is needed. This may also be true if the negative self-talk is keeping you isolated and avoiding relationships.

Here is my theory on stressors. Imagine this metaphor if you find yourself feeling and thinking: "This isn't me! I can't do anything right and I hate myself."

> If I asked you to walk up a big hill, and no matter what I did, I told you, you had to keep walking in order to feel better. I then had you throw a gunnysack over your back, and as you walked, I would start to put boulders in it. There will be a point when no matter how motivated you were, you would be unable to keep walking because of the weight of the sack.
>
> Compare the stressors to the boulders. Our minds and bodies eventually get to the point of *enough*, where the body or the mind starts to shut down and we need to ask for help. There are situations that no one is prepared for, and we all have times in our lives where we are over-whelmed. Remember, it's OK to ask for help!

If you find that you have tried to stop the *judge (voice chattering at you)* and can't, you might want to check in with a therapist or a psychiatrist. Remember, you deserve to feel good about yourself. ***You count.***

A man needs self-acceptance
or he can't live with himself;
he needs self-criticism
or others can't live with him.
—James A. Pike, American minister (1913-1969)

Chapter 9

Commitment to Stay in the Present

Nothing is worth more than this day.
—Johann Wolfgang Goethe, German poet (1749-1832)

Just for today, what would be *good enough*? Using that term throughout this book, my hope is that it helps you stay away from the *what if's* and the *if only's*. How often do you tempt yourself with: "*What if* I won the lottery?" "*What if* they don't like my presentation?" "*What if* I drive all the way over and they are closed?" It's OK to fantasize, but if you are spending a good part of your salary on lottery tickets or going to the worst-case scenario, you need to read this chapter.

I frequently hear "*If only* I lost those 25 pounds, I would _____." There are multiple ways to end that sentence. It may include: "get a boyfriend," "be less self conscious," "quit yelling at myself about my weight," or "stop feeling guilty about what I eat." When asked, "Is it a possibility it will happen before the end of the day?" they usually will smile and say "No." Then we get to work deciding what tools they need to "commit to stay in the moment and value today."

I used to think that when I graduated from medical school, I would have it made. Then it became, "*When* I finish my residency, I'll have it made." I figured that if I had all my training behind me, the pressure would be off. Wrong! Can you see where this thinking was leading me? I didn't take the time to identify those things happening during my day that gave my life value and meaning.

Sure, it was exciting to deliver a baby or learn a new procedure, yet the *if only's* would pop up again.

This lesson deepened when looking to apply to a residency in psychiatry. I was getting frantic about making the right choice and was filled with the *what if's*! *What if* I don't get time with the attending, *what if* I only have six months of wards instead of eight months, *what if* I don't like the other residents, *what if* I can't find an apartment, *what if* it isn't the program I thought it would be, *what if* I am not as good as the other residents?

My residency director recognized the signs and asked me to come talk to her. She pointed out that I was driving myself nuts trying to pick the *perfect program*; and that the worst case scenario would be that, if after my internship year I decided that it wasn't a good fit, I could transfer to another program. This took the pressure off, and I was able to enjoy the final months of medical school. I almost lost out on the fun and the excitement of watching my goal of becoming a doctor get closer and closer. It taught me a valuable lesson.

What is keeping you from making the commitment to staying in the moment and making the most of your day?

Do any of us have guarantees that we'll be around for another day? NO! I'm sure all of you have heard the "live as each day is your last one" proposition, yet how many of us do that? We get so wrapped up in our daily routine that it isn't until we lose someone close or hear about a tragedy that we consider our own mortality.

When I work with people with anorexia who are filled with pain and fear, I'll ask them to imagine waking up without their disease. Several questions are posed: "Who would notice first?" "What would you do differently?"

Write down three people who would first recognize that you were different in your approach to the day if you made an effort to focus on the day.

1._____

2._____

3._____

Did you try in some way to make today yours? Which of the following suggestions make sense?

- Take extra time with your kids or animals.

- Watch the sunset.

- Prepare a special meal: it can be simple but something you really enjoy.

- Smile at more people.

- Smell a flower.

- Make a phone call to someone you really enjoy talking to.

- Give yourself an affirmation.

- Say a quick prayer.

- Others: _____

- _____

- _____

The list could go on and on, but you get the idea.

**Yesterday is gone and tomorrow has not yet come.
We must live each day as if it were our last.**
—Mother Teresa, Indian humanitarian (1910-1997)

One of the tasks of the elderly is to look back over their lives and make some sort of *peace* with it. Are they satisfied or was it *good enough*? Can they go back and change things? Of course not, so why not make peace with what time they have left? I would hate to be remembered as *the angry person* or *the bitter person* by my loved ones.

How do you go about committing to stay in the present moment? People in recovery use the idea of giving up those things that they can't control and focusing on what they can *(The Serenity Prayer)*. It is a way of grounding yourself and admitting to yourself that there are some things you need to let go of in order to enjoy your day.

In Chapter 1, I talked about using the **Daily Psychological Inventory** to get in touch with feelings that you are hanging onto from the previous day, week or decade.

Do you know people who are *carrying a grudge* or families who have members who aren't speaking to one another? Incongruently, people's words "I don't want to waste my energy on so and so" often does not match their behaviors, and I have a ringside seat to their anger as they describe the situation.

Does that take energy? Yep. Are they going to hold onto it for the rest of their lives? We frequently work on letting go of anger or hurt in order to focus on what they want to focus on to stay in the moment. If you dwell on the past, you stay stuck; and if you worry about tomorrow, it is easy to miss out on today.

List two things that you can focus on just for today?

1._____

2._____

List two things that you worry about in the future that you are willing to *commit to letting go* in order to focus on today.

1._____

2._____

Does worrying ever serve you? Some could argue that it is a form of anxiety that keeps you on your toes so the unexpected doesn't catch you off guard; but more often, the opposite is true. Do you have fears that run over and over again in your head that you wish you could let go, block out, and quit thinking about?

It takes practice to *let things go*. If you have perfected the *art of worrying*, begin by working with the small things.

Ask yourself what the worst-case scenario would be if

_____.

Then decide if it is worth the effort. Go for it. Worry until you can't think about it anymore. If the worst-case scenario is not a life-or-death situation, give it reasonable time, and then move on.

Say to yourself: "What is the worst that will happen if I don't get the job" or "if I don't get pregnant this month" or "if I splurge on a purchase?" Is someone going to shoot you? *(I don't think so.)*

Start by putting things in perspective. Pick your battles and concentrate on winning the war by quieting *the worry monster* (as a colleague calls it). Focus on your priorities for the day and see how you can *take action* to make the most out of today.

A woman went into the hospital to have a routine procedure, a D & C. Knowing she would be *put under*, she had a *worry monster attack*! After reading Dale Carnegie's book, HOW TO STOP WORRYING AND START LIVING, while waiting for the surgery, she did the exercise, "What is the worst thing that will happen?"

Over thirty years later, she recalls the incident with rare clarity. Her worst fear was that she would die under anesthetic. Asking herself what the statistics were that that would happen, she crossed that worry off her list. Doing the same with each worry, by the time she went into surgery, she was very relaxed without a single worry left in her mind.

Once out of surgery, she felt no pain and decided to take a walk down the hospital hallway. She got to the nurse's station to ask a question, and suddenly she got faint and had to sit down.

The nurse exclaimed: "What are you doing out of bed? You aren't supposed to be walking! You just came out of anesthetic! Didn't you know we had those guardrails up for a reason? You get right back to bed!"

Giggling to herself, she thought that she was so successful at being stress-free that she had a D & C without any discomfort or even awareness that she needed rest and recuperation time afterwards!

Several patients come in just to get help with problem solving. "I just don't think of those things," a patient will tell me.

Worried that she would get lost trying to find a new meeting place her friends had picked, she got so anxious that she considered canceling the lunch even though she had been looking forward to it.

When asked what she could do to ease her anxiety and take control, she struggled to come up with an idea. "What if you use your cell phone when you know you are close and have them talk you into *landing correctly,* or take a cab?"

She smiled and agreed; she could let go of the *what-if thinking* and take one of those actions.

My uncle made the statement *(and I am I sure wasn't the first to hear it)* when he was asked if he wanted to plan a trip, "I don't even buy green bananas!" I laughed and realized he has learned to stay in the moment.

As we age, this sometimes gets harder to do as our lives get more complex or health problems limit our options. It takes courage to give up some dreams when worried about the future, especially if you know realistically that there will be a difficult path ahead. Yet, what does the worry do for you?

It is OK to get help from a therapist or those organizations that are set up to help people deal with problems associated with aging. Have you met those that you know are *young at heart* and seem ageless?

It is a lot easier to commit to stay in the day if you can focus on what you have rather than don't have, or what you can do rather than what you can't do. I help patients grieve the loss of those things that are out of their reach and allow them to have their anger, sadness, bargaining, denial and acceptance (stages of grief). We then start planning ways to make these losses tolerable and move on.

If you are the type of person that can't tolerate not knowing what is coming next, then go ahead and make some short term, intermediate and long term goals; but remember to make them manageable.

For example, if I decide that I am going to see thirty patients every day, then I am setting myself up. If I decide that I will see at least one therapy patient a day *(something I really enjoy)*, then that is a manageable goal. My intermediate goal may be to increase the number of therapy patients I see each day, and my long-term goal may be just to do therapy and no medication management.

Think about what is important to help you commit to stay in your day. Is it good enough to work out for a half an hour if you know that you will be late if you try to take more time? Then give yourself permission to totally enjoy that half hour.

> A patient likes to push herself when riding her bike. I helped her give up the *hard runs* when she knew deep down that her body was tired, or it would not serve her to push it. She learned to enjoy the less trying rides. She was still out in the fresh air doing something she loved to do. Instead of getting frustrated, she could stay in the moment and just enjoy.

Can you relate to something you strive for that could be done on a lesser level and still be *good enough*? I am not talking about compromising your goals—just about not setting your standards so high that you take the ability to enjoy the moment out of the picture.

List three things that you worry about that you *can't* resolve today. **(This is different than the above exercise.)**

1._____

2._____

3._____

List three things that you commit to and *need* to get done today.
(This is also different than the above exercise: *need* and *want* are
two different concepts.)

1._____

2._____

3._____

Do the "worst case scenario" reasoning on these three commitments and notice what the consequences would be if you did not
do them today. Your commitments to do what you can each day
prevent you from having things happen in your life that you don't
want or need. Taking action on your commitments is a great
antidote to worry!

I'm not saying that you can't anticipate and enjoy upcoming
plans or events. It is when you can't get done what you need to
because you are *stuck* in the anticipatory anxiety, fear, or anger. For
example, if you can't think of anything except for getting your
taxes done, and you can't possible complete them until you get
further forms back, you will be wasting your energy on something
you can't control.

A common problem is when people go through a long drawn-
out divorce and get stuck in the "what if they do this" mode. It takes
them out of the moment and sabotages the day.

EXERCISE:

Imagine committing to stay in the moment and see how it feels.

• Are you feeling less stressed?

- Do you find yourself being aware of what you were feeling and thinking?

- Are you able to focus better and feel settled?

Keep practicing and it will come. The more times you actually bask in the present moment, the more those moments will multiply.

Each moment is precious and unrecoverable.
—Jon Kabat-Zinn, American psychologist

Chapter 10

Commitment to Give Back
What I Have Learned

This is our purpose:
to make as meaningful as possible this life
to live in such a way that we may be proud of ourselves;
to act in such a way that some part of us lives on.
—Oswald Spengler, German philosopher (1880-1936)

I recently had the privilege to meet someone who had been through two terrible accidents and was now doing inspirational speaking. He had suffered a broken neck, was in rehabilitation, and managed to get well enough to be released. Then he was in another car accident that put him back to square one. The pain and suffering he endured was almost beyond belief. He was left paralyzed and in a wheelchair. I thought his talk was going to be about regaining his spirituality. It was in a way, but the amazing thing was his gift of humor and honesty that left me questioning what I could do to *give back* from some of the experiences I've had in learning about mental illness and recovery. Here was someone who had every right to be angry and hateful, yet he shared his gratitude at being allowed to speak to us that night. His courage and ability to go beyond his own suffering was truly inspiring.

Some of you may think it is easy if you are in the position of therapist or psychiatrist *to give back what you have learned*—and even better that we get paid to do it! I am not talking about repeating *pearls* that can improve behavior and outcomes.

This chapter is about **being the role model of behaviors for those around you who can benefit from the changes you chose to make.**

Is anger something you need to work on? Would your family describe you as a *rager*? It would probably come as no surprise if you took the first step towards controlling that behavior to see family members notice and adjust their behavior.

Some moms and dads are full of shame and guilt because they have yelled at their kids when they felt out of control and couldn't stop themselves or walk away at the moment. When they learn to control their anger, they give their family a priceless gift.

To start the change process and improve your relationships, ask yourself this question *prior* to speaking: "Is what I am about to say going to benefit that person, or is it *my stuff* that I need to hear myself speak?" Can you imagine how that would cut down on the amount of unnecessary conversation? Hopefully, it would also decrease the number of things said that hurt, scare, frustrate, belittle and embarrass others.

How many times have you wanted to *take back something* you have said? There are things we said that are also misinterpreted because we didn't stop to consider how they would be perceived.

A colleague lectured about how we are so reactive to the word *fat*. Half listening, I heard him say, "Dr. Berkus, you're looking fat today!" He was doing it to make his point, but I joked with him afterward that he caught me off guard, and it would take years of therapy now to get past that remark. His point was that he could have said that I looked healthy or fit or well, and my response would have been different. **(Definitely!)** He said what he did to get a deliberate reaction, but what about the things that are said without realizing how damaging they can be to someone?

At the theater, I heard a mom berating her son who was about ten years old. She kept asking him over and over again why he didn't go to the restroom with her when she asked him to ten minutes before. So here is this child being shamed in front of a group of people and still having to use the restroom. She kept asking the *why* questions. Since he was bright, he could have come up with a number of *because* answers *(as a therapist once explained to me),* but what didn't change was the fact that he still *had to go* before the end of intermission. Mom chose to stay stuck in the *why's* and not in what needed the energy at the moment *(get the kid some relief!).*

Do you find yourself asking a lot of *why's?* Have you become great at *because* answers. Do the answers change anything? Frequently patients say, "Why did my dad leave us?" "Why couldn't they show more love?"

We can focus our time on getting *because* answers, or we could move on and work on what *in the moment* needs our attention.

It is fun for me to hear when my patients have changed their behavior and are now able to function much more effectively and *give back*, whether it is to another person, job, or society. I will frequently ask, "Who is noticing the changes in your behavior?" Most of the time the answers will be "my spouse" or "my parents" or "my kids."

The other response is "I'm the person I want to be" in contrast to what they were when they were mentally unfit. "I wish I would have gotten help years ago!" (Watch out for the *if only's.*) Sometimes people don't realize how bad they were really feeling until it got better. "I can't believe I can feel this way" is fun to hear from someone who has had their ADHD (attention deficit hyperactivity disorder) treated or their co-dependency explained and addressed.

It may be hard for them at first because the *rules* are changing. If you have been the one to try meet the needs of others *(expecting payback)* and find yourself angry and resentful, then learn to set healthy boundaries so the other people in your life begin to *get it* that you are getting mentally healthier. It may mean they have to start meeting their own needs, which can cause some feelings. That's OK. Keep talking to them about it. It isn't them that you are reacting to—it's their behavior.

It's similar to one person choosing to eat healthy foods while the rest of the family wants to stay stuck with the junk food. They may know it is time for a change but find it hard to watch you be the one to actually make the needed changes. As you feel and look better as a result of your choices, they may decide to change their behaviors, especially if your new boundary is to buy only healthy foods. Change is hard and we are set up to *keep the status quo* even if it isn't serving us anymore.

The take-home message of this commitment to give back is that if you are feeling better about yourself and your behavior, it will spill into many areas of your life. You may now have a new appreciation of what people can mean in your life and reach out more. Giving back may look like passing this book to someone who is struggling with the boundary of your role of being a friend (or relative), *not their therapist*. You are just a concerned person who identifies that they need help.

Let's pretend that you walk away from reading this book with the idea that you are going to behave in a way that you know is the right way to behave. There is no other motive. You may start to find yourself picking up a piece of trash or giving back too much change given by a sales person. NO ONE IS GOING TO CLAP.

Is it *good enough* if it brings a smile to your face or to give yourself a pat on the back? Sure. Watch it spill over into the workplace, home, time with friends, animals, and your kids. You'll find that type of giving back can help you feel better and focus on that glass half full.

Hopefully, you will start to observe your behavior more often rather than just reacting to a situation; and your commitment to taking action will bring a sign of relief and reduce the negative feelings you have been having in regards to yourself.

Remember, the major question you can keep asking yourself over and over is: "Is my way working?" If the answer is "no," you know you can keep working on yourself.

You may get into the habit of asking yourself if your behavior is the *same old same old* or did you just choose to react differently.

Was it hard? Did it feel strange? Did you consider other options?

By now, you have gained some insight and son of a gun if you aren't noticing other people's poor mental health. Are you tempted to intervene? DON'T! Just agree to keep monitoring your own feelings, choices, needs, responses, and actions.

Life is too short to be in constant poor mental health. There are too many consequences. Give yourself permission to make the commitments and start to like yourself and your behavior, maybe for the first time in a long time. YOU DESERVE TO FEEL MENTALLY FIT!

Now that you have make it through all the Ten Commitments, ask yourself, "What made sense for you? What fit?" In order to start to give back, you may want to complete this chart to see how you want to set up your new priorities.

Benefits of Being Physically Fit Benefits of Being Mentally Fit

Still not real motivated? How about completing this chart?

Consequences of being mentally unfit

Are you willing to stay with your current behaviors and experience the consequences? How about looking at Commitment One again. It might help you decide to make some short-term goals in changing your thoughts, feelings, and behaviors.

Your day will pass, so why not make it a great one instead of *just another day*. Did you ever notice how a stranger smiling and acknowledging you can feel good? Well, if each of us smiled at someone just because we can, and it doesn't cost us a lot, why not make the commitment to be an active participant in your day. Notice, acknowledge, share good feelings, and *give back* because *you count* and can make a difference in your day and someone else's.

Afterword

An unexamined life is not worth living.
—Socrates, Greek philosopher (B.C. 469–399)

Congratulations! If you are reading this, it hopefully means that you have made it through the **Ten Commitments** and hopefully you are talking to yourself. (Sometimes it is healthy to do that.) I know it is a lot to take in.

Keep what makes sense and fits for you.
Let go what doesn't.

The Talmud teaches that when you are willing to learn, a teacher will appear. This book could have been titled: EVERYTHING I NEEDED TO LEARN, I LEARNED IN MEDICAL SCHOOL. That is not the whole truth: my patients were the *real books*, just as the psychiatrist in medical school taught us would be the case. Using this information he so wonderfully taught has been the basis in my practice and hopefully in being mentally fit. Amazingly, after almost 13 years, his words are with me on a daily basis and appear throughout this book. I don't know where he is, but I will always be grateful for his dedication to his students.

My hope is that TEN COMMITMENTS TO MENTAL FITNESS has increased your awareness. If you choose to change one behavior, then it has been worth it. Please know that all of us can continue to choose to learn, better our understanding of our behavior, and gain self-awareness as to how it affects those lives we touch.

Just as there are rewards to being physically fit, you will find rewards in becoming mentally fit. It is a process and can take time. The time will pass anyway, so why not put it to good use.

After fifteen years of studying and treating mental illness, I wanted to contribute to promoting mental fitness. I have learned by watching my patients get well how precious it is to have your mental fitness. My heart goes out to those who struggle on a daily basis. This is my small way of *giving back*. Now I can honestly answer patients who ask in their pain:

"Why does it have to be this way?"

It doesn't.

AFFIRMATIONS FOR MENTAL FITNESS

1. COMMITMENT TO KNOW I COUNT
I count, my thoughts count, and my feelings count!

2. COMMITMENT TO
TAKE RESPONSIBILITY FOR MY FEELINGS
I have a variety of feelings. I act on them in healthy ways.

3. COMMITMENT TO SET PRIORITIES IN MY LIFE
I know what is most important to me
and set my goals accordingly.

4. COMMITMENT TO WORK ON MY CURRENT
RELATIONSHIPS AND ROLES
I value my relationships
and work on honesty and appreciation to enrich them.

5. COMMITMENT TO SET HEALTHY BOUNDARIES
I decide which roles I feel obligated to take on
and which roles I want to take on willingly.

6. COMMITMENT TO GROW SPIRITUALLY
I honor my humanness and
use my abilities to spiritually grow.

7. COMMITMENT TO IDENTIFY
MY MIND-BODY CONNECTION
I honor all my basis needs:
sleep, exercise, nutrition, and support.

8. COMMITMENT TO CHANGE MY SELF-TALK
I treat myself with love and respect.

9. COMMITMENT TO STAY IN THE PRESENT
I stop and consider what I can let go of
and what I can control.

10. COMMITMENT TO GIVE BACK WHAT I HAVE LEARNED
I work to make my presence meaningful.

NOTES: